DISCARD

THE
PLANT
PARADOX
FAMILY
COOKBOOK

THE PLANT PARADOX FAMILY COOKBOOK

80 One-Pot Recipes to Nourish Your Family Using Your
Instant Pot, Slow Cooker, or Sheet Pan

STEVEN R. GUNDRY, MD

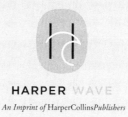

HARPER WAVE

An Imprint of HarperCollinsPublishers

FIRST EDITION

Produced by Stonesong Press, LLC
Designed by Andy Taray, Ohioboy Design Co.
Photographs by Evi Abeler
page ix: Photograph by Cookie Schulte, © 2018

Library of Congress Cataloging-in-Publication Data has been applied for.

ISBN 978-0-06-291183-4

19 20 21 22 23   LSC   10 9 8 7 6 5 4 3 2 1

Dedication

To our daughters Elizabeth and Melissa, their husbands Tim and Ray, and our grand-children, Sophie and Oliver, all who demonstrate daily the benefits of the Plant Paradox Program on themselves and their families.

CONTENTS

Introduction

On the surface, it may seem unusual for a heart surgeon and cardiologist to write a cookbook for families. After all, most cardiologists tend to treat adult patients, often those of advanced age. But what many people don't know is that back when I was a Professor of Surgery at Loma Linda University School of Medicine, I was also a Professor of Pediatrics and a Fellow of the American Academy of Pediatrics (AAP). In addition to seeing my cardiac patients, I also see a great number of families in my current practices in Palm Springs and Santa Barbara, California. Most of the children and young adults I see are suffering from an autoimmune disease that has defied traditional treatments. Other times, my younger patients are brought in by a parent who has regained his or her own health by following my nutritional protocol, and are hopeful their child or children can benefit similarly.

These parents come to see me with a lot of questions, and no small amount of concern about feeding their children a diet that is contrary to what their pediatricians have advised, or even what AAP suggests is optimal. After all, we are told to feed our children cow's milk, grains, fruit, and legumes from their first birthday onward. The idea that such foods could be harmful—as I suggest in *The Plant Paradox* and my subsequent books—causes parents no small amount of worry. They come to me looking for advice and explanation, wanting to better understand how their children can follow my protocol safely.

In addition, ever since the publication of *The Plant Paradox Cookbook*, I've received thousands of emails and messages from readers asking how they can make my recipes more suitable for their families—and asking for recipes that can be thrown together quickly, without a lot of complicated cooking or difficult-to-find ingredients. These are people who have had success on the Plant Paradox program and are eager to cook nutritious meals everyone in their family will enjoy. They are parents of kids who have turned around their autoimmune diseases and gone off immunosuppressive drugs, who are finding it challenging to keep their child's progress on track for the long run. They are also, very often, working moms and dads who have little to no time to cook every night of the week, and are on a food budget that doesn't allow for lots of fancy ingredients.

The Plant Paradox Family Cookbook is written, first and foremost, with the needs of these patients and readers in mind, as well as for all of you who have successfully followed the Plant Paradox program and restored your health, but wonder: *How do I make this a sustainable lifestyle with a family*

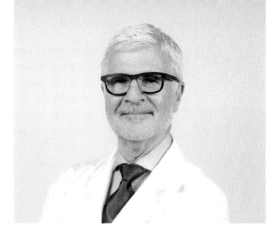

to cook and care for? And perhaps equally important, *How can I make sure my kids are getting all the nutrients they need?*

Well, dear reader, you have come to the right place. This cookbook is designed to give answers to these questions and more. I want to make the Plant Paradox program a lifestyle you and your family can live with, literally and figuratively.

The reality is that the Plant Paradox plan is a way of eating that works for everyone, regardless of age. It's that simple. I've documented the positive changes in the bloodwork of thousands of patients in my clinics. I've seen diabetic kids reverse their diabetes, obese kids slim down, skinny kids put on some much-needed weight for the first time in their lives, and yes, reversed autoimmune diseases, reversed asthma, eczema, and even cystic acne. I've reported these results and more at major national and international meetings, but the real joy I get is when I receive an email, a letter, or read a review online that shares your positive experiences with the program and your amazing successes.

Finally, this book is also written for all the "holdouts" who have heard about this crazy Plant Paradox thing—that some plants are out to kill us or at least hurt us, and that the traditional mainstays of a "healthy" diet like whole grains, low-fat dairy, and legumes are actually some of the worst foods we can consume. Maybe you've been skeptical of my approach, or maybe you've read through the guidelines and simply thought, "that's not for me." I understand that change is hard, and I would ask you to consider this: changing your diet and lifestyle doesn't only affect your health. It affects the health and long-term wellbeing of your whole family. My intention with this book is to make it as easy and enjoyable as possible to adapt a healthier lifestyle for every member of your family, without needing to give up the foods and traditions you and your loved ones enjoy. You can still have pizza night, still eat spaghetti and meatballs, pack a sandwich for school lunches, indulge in an ice pop on a hot sunny day. You can celebrate food and enjoy family meals together that are fuss-free, quick to assemble, and provide the very best nutrition for the people you love.

Everything you need is in these pages. If you haven't read *The Plant Paradox* or my other books, not to worry—I'm going to offer a brief overview of the protocol here so you can jump right in and join the club. Over the next few chapters, we'll take a closer look at the nutritional needs of kids as well as the basics of the Plant Paradox lifestyle so all of us, old hands or newbies alike, can quickly get up to speed before diving into the kitchen. Welcome to *The Plant Paradox Family Cookbook!*

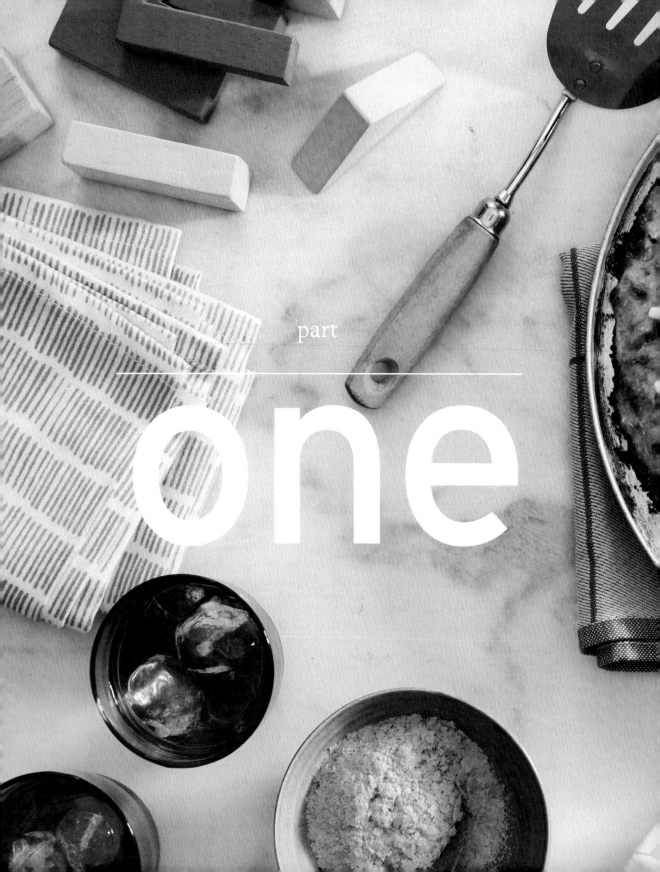

part

one

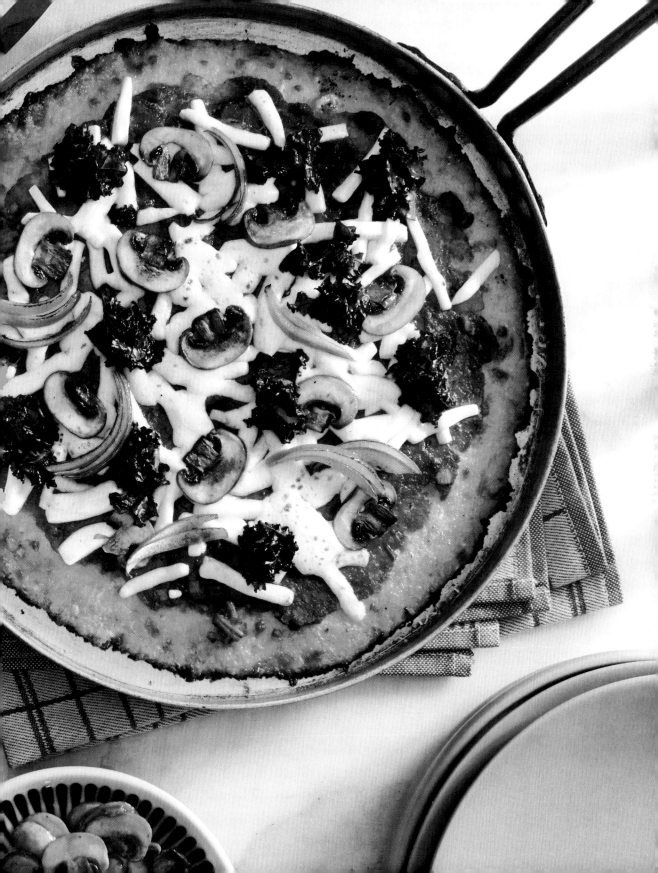

chapter one

Lectins and
Your Health

In my first cookbook, I opened with these wise words from Michael Pollan's elegant start to *The Omnivore's Dilemma*: "Eat food. Not too much. Mostly plants."

In essence, I couldn't agree more with this sentiment. A plant-based diet is certainly better for our health than one comprised of poor-quality animal protein and processed foods. But contrary to what many of us have been taught, not all plants are good for us. And in fact, some can be downright harmful to our health—in particular, those that contain a high concentration of proteins called lectins.

And therein lies the paradox: plants can be both friend and enemy, good and bad, nutritious and disease-promoting.

It's likely that some of the foods you've long considered the healthiest for you, and certainly, for your children, are actually those that contain a high concentration of lectins. These foods include most grains, beans and other legumes; certain nuts and seeds; and many fruits, as well as most vegetables with seeds, such as tomatoes, cucumbers, and eggplant (which are botanically fruit).

I know it can feel confusing and contradictory to learn that the foods you've relied on as the cornerstone of a healthy lifestyle are actually undermining your and your family's wellness. So before we go any further we're going to take a closer look at lectins—what they are, what they do, and why you should avoid them.

Predator and Prey

Let's go back some 450 million years, to a time when plants reigned supreme as the only living organisms on the planet. This was the golden age for plants—they had no predators, and plenty of sunlight and precipitation to grow and proliferate. Now, fast forward about 100 million years, when insects and later, animals, arrive on the scene. What do they want to eat? Plants! But like all living things, plants have an imperative to grow, reproduce, and, well, not die—survival is encoded in their DNA. So they adapted to their new environment, developing short- and long-term defense strategies to protect themselves from predators. These short-term defense strategies included poisoning, paralyzing, or entrapping their predators to cease an attack immediately. Their long-term defense strategy? Producing chemicals that sicken their enemy, little by little, eventually debilitating them.

As you might have guessed, lectins are part of a plant's long-term defense strategy. Lectins are present in all plants, but are highly concentrated in only a few—such as nightshades (tomatoes, eggplant, peppers, potatoes), most grains, legumes, and many fruits. The skins and seeds of plants contain the greatest density of lectins. Why the seeds? Well, plants have an imperative not only to survive themselves, but also to ensure their offspring (aka seeds) survive. Fruit-bearing plants have a special trick to protect their offspring and ensure proliferation: As the fruit ripens, its lectin concentration decreases. When a fruit is fully ripe, its seeds are able to pass through an animal's digestive system intact and are excreted out, where they end up in the soil to begin new life. But when the fruit is unripe, the lectins in those seeds—which are not yet fully mature, and thus cannot generate new life once deposited in the soil—wreak havoc in the digestive tract of the animal that consumes them. Hopefully this animal learns its lesson after a few belly aches: only eat the fruit when it is fully ripe.

So, what about those belly aches, then? How do lectins do their damage inside the body? To better understand this, it's helpful to take a brief tour of the GI system. Your digestive tract (aka, your intestines, or your "gut"), is a labyrinthine tunnel filled with many twists and turns. If it were all stretched out and laid flat, it could cover a tennis court. The job of your digestive system is to process the foods you eat (to "digest" them), and break them down into their essential components. Your body extracts the nutrients it can use, including amino acids from the protein you eat, sugar molecules from carbohydrates, and fatty acids from fats. If everything is working as it should, eventually these molecules make their way outside of your gut and are transported via your bloodstream to be absorbed by the cells that need them. But the other components of your food—the waste, the toxins, the indigestible fiber—stay inside the walls until they are eventually excreted.

A good analogy is to think of your gut like a tunnel you drive through to cross a river. When you're in the tunnel, you're surrounded by water, but it is safely contained on the other side of the tunnel's wall. Similarly, the food that travels through your digestive tract is encased in a "tunnel" of sorts. Any food particles that enter that tunnel aren't technically part of your body, where your circulatory system functions as the river rushing through. They stay inside the tube, protected by the gut wall.

While the surface area of your intestines is vast, the gut wall itself is quite fragile—it is just one cell thick. The cells that make up this barrier are lined up neatly side by side, connected to one another by impenetrable seals known as "tight junctions." These tight junctions function as gatekeepers that decide what passes through the wall, and what stays inside. Normally, the only molecules able to pass through these gates are the nutrients your body needs, which happen to be very small molecules.

As an extra layer of protection, this single layer of cells also produces mucus, made of polysaccharides (complex sugars), to entrap any rogue molecules that may try to make their way out of the gut and into the bloodstream. Lectins are sticky proteins that easily bind to specific sugar molecules—including, but not exclusively, the polysaccharides that make up this mucus layer. Once inside your gut, they find these polysaccharides and attach themselves to them.

Now, if you have a healthy gut wall protected by a thick layer of mucus, the lectins get stuck, can't make it through the tight junctions, and that's the end of it. But if your mucus layer is thin, or if your diet is heavy in lectin-containing foods, or you've been exposed to a group of toxins I call the 7 Deadly Disruptors (more on that soon), those lectins will get to the target they really came for. Attaching to your single-cell wall, they flip a chemical switch that breaks apart the tight junctions. Wham! The cells pull apart, and lectins push right on through the wall and into your bloodstream. Over time, lectins begin to damage the gut wall, creating microscopic holes that cause other molecules to continuously leak out—a condition commonly known as "leaky gut syndrome."

The integrity of your gut wall is so important to your health that your body places a lot of resources nearby to protect it: about 65 percent of your immune system's white blood cells are amassed there, just waiting to be called into action. What does that "action" look like, when it comes to defending the wall? In a word: inflammation. Think about what happens when your immune system responds to an invader externally—for example, when you get a splinter in your finger. The whole area around the splinter becomes red and swollen, right? That's because the splinter is a foreign substance; the redness and swelling of your skin is a result of your white blood cells attacking the invader. Similarly, when lectins make their way outside the tunnel of your GI tract, they become like "splinters." Once in the bloodstream, your immune system quickly identifies lectins as intruders and initiates an inflammatory response to protect you from harm. In addition to lectins, your immune system also monitors to make sure the bacteria in your gut stay on their side of the wall. But trillions of bacteria grow and reproduce and die daily, producing smaller bits of cell debris that can also leak outside of the gut once the wall contains holes. These dead bacterial cell walls are called lipopolysaccharides, or LPSs. Your immune system cannot tell the difference between the cell wall of a dead bacteria or a live one, so if an LPS gets loose in your bloodstream, further inflammation is generated.

When this immune response takes place regularly—as is the case if lectins are breaking down your gut wall—you can develop a chronic condition in which the immune system becomes so upregulated and hypervigilant that it begins to attack even healthy cells that, on the surface, pose no threat. This is known as autoimmunity. I sometimes refer to autoimmunity as "friendly fire," in which the body targets the good guys—which could be anything from skin cells to thyroid cells to nerve cells—by mistake. Common autoimmune diseases include rheumatoid arthritis, Crohn's disease, lupus, Hashimoto's disease, multiple sclerosis, Grave's disease, celiac disease, vitiligo, psoriasis, IBS, and type-1 diabetes. More than 70 percent of my practice now is devoted to treating patients—including a large number of children—who suffer from autoimmune diseases. Thankfully, most of these patients are able to reverse their autoimmune illnesses simply by removing lectins from their diet. By avoiding or neutralizing lectins in your food, you remove a root cause of autoimmunity and give your gut a chance to heal.

The Silent Majority

Okay, so we've covered the basic biology and function of the gut, and you understand how lectins can trigger chronic inflammation. But there's another way that lectins cause major dysfunction in the gut: by harming the trillions of inhabitants that reside there. I'm talking about your gut bacteria, also known as your microbiome.

The microorganisms that live in your gut help to digest food and extract nutrients from it, protect you from pathogens (bacteria and other dangerous bugs), and play a role in regulating everything from your metabolism to your mood to your immune system. I like to call these microbes our "gut buddies," because they do so many beneficial things for us—in fact, they are so essential to our health that we literally could not live without them.

As we evolved, so did our microbiome. When our diet consisted primarily of foraged plants and tubers—along with some occasional animal protein, particularly shellfish and fish—our gut buddies thrived and evolved the ability to digest the lectins in these foods. They also "taught" our immune system, via chemical messages, that certain common lectins held no threat, and there was no need for our bodies to respond to these foods with inflammation. But after the last Ice Age ended, about 10,000 years ago, we had to find new food sources, as most plants and animals that we'd long relied on for sustenance had died out. And so, we learned how to cultivate crops: mainly grains and beans, which were able to be dried and stored—an asset that made them highly valuable.

Instead of spending most of our time foraging for food, we were able to cultivate shelf-stable foods, domesticate animals, and shift our focus on creating a more "developed" society. But where we made advances in language, philosophy, and infrastructure, we lost ground when it came to our nutrition. With the introduction of these crops also came the introduction of novel lectins into our diet—lectins our bodies, and specifically, our gut buddies, weren't equipped to digest. And while you might think that the last ten thousand years should've bought us, and the microbes that live within us, enough time to evolve the ability to handle these lectins, the reality is that such a timespan is a blink in evolutionary terms. We weren't prepared to properly digest these new lectins then, and thanks to changes in our food supply and environment, we are even less prepared to digest them now.

Gut Bugs and The Brain

Recent research has confirmed that the health of the microbiome directly impacts mental health and behavior in children. Researchers at Arizona State University used a method called fecal transplantation—in which the microbes of a healthy person are transferred to an individual with a less healthy microbiome—to study the effects of microbial transfer for children with autism spectrum disorder, or ASD. (It is not uncommon for children with ASD to experience gastrointestinal problems.)

The researchers found that not only did the children's GI and behavioral symptoms dramatically improve following the treatment, but also that the positive effects endured over time. Two years following treatment, the initial improvements in gut symptoms remained and a whopping 45 percent reduction in ASD symptoms (including speech, social interaction, behavior) was observed.[1]

In my practice, I've also been thrilled to witness symptoms alleviate for children who suffer from anxiety and depression once we get their nutrition right and start healing their gut. Even if your child has not been diagnosed with a specific mental health or cognitive issue, don't be surprised if you notice improvements in his or her overall mood and mental acuity when their gut health is restored. A healthier gut makes for a less inflamed brain—and that's good for everyone's health.

Our Changing Diet

Clearly, humans have been eating lectin-containing foods for millions of years. So, you might rightly wonder: Why is it that we only now seem to be experiencing their negative effects?

One reason is that early humans simply ate fewer lectin-rich plants than we do today. Remember, the advent of agriculture and all of those storable grains and legumes is a relatively new component of our diet. Additional trials came with the introduction of foods originating in the Americas, also known as the "New World." These crops included corn, squash, tomatoes, potatoes, peppers, quinoa, and other "healthy" mainstays of the typical American diet. While populations native to the continent—the Native Americans—had up to fifteen thousand years of exposure to these plants and prepared them in ways that reduced their lectin content, those "new" to consuming them—populations from Africa, Europe, and Asia—have had less than five hundred years of exposure.

More recently, our diet has changed in other ways. Over the last several decades, fruits and vegetables that were once eaten seasonally have become available year-round. Want blueberries in November or tomatoes in February? You can find them, imported from Chile or Mexico, now permanently occupying a shelf in your local grocery store. Eating out-of-season fruit, which is harvested before it is ripe (and thus contains more lectins than normally ripened fruits), shipped thousands of miles away, and then artificially ripened with ethylene gas, unwittingly exposes you and your children to a huge amount of gut-busting lectins.

Another recent change to our diet is that over the last half century or so, we've come to rely on processed foods, typically made from high-lectin ingredients such as wheat, corn, soy, and vegetable oils. And even if you've been studiously avoiding processed foods over concerns for your health, misinformation about nutrition has likely steered you toward "healthy" foods—like tofu, brown rice, whole grains, and low-fat dairy products—that are actually terrible for your health and full of lectins. At the same time, we've decreased our intake of the types of foods our gut buddies thrive on—fermented vegetables, tubers, and cruciferous vegetables.

The animals we eat also contribute to our modern health problems. For starters, we eat much more animal protein now than our ancestors ever did, despite what you may have heard about "caveman" diets. In addition, the quality of that protein has changed radically. Today the majority of the animals we eat are raised on industrial lots where they are fed a diet of corn- and soy-based feed. This lectin-rich diet causes so many digestive problems for the animals that ranchers douse the feed with calcium carbonate—the active ingredient in the antacids humans take. As you've heard me say, you are what you eat. And when it comes to eating animal products, you are what the thing you are eating, ate. Consuming lectins indirectly through meat, eggs, and dairy harms the gut wall, wipes out your gut buddies, and keeps your immune system continuously activated, instigating chronic inflammation.

The Ancient Instant Pot

Believe it or not, a crude bonfire and a trendy pressure cooker have more in common you might expect. When humans discovered fire, and the ability to control it, they gained two advantages: the ability to stay warm, and the ability to cook food. Applying heat to food was a game-changer—not only did cooking food make it taste better, it also made it easier to digest.

That's because cooking breaks down the cell walls of plants, which are otherwise indigestible. This is even true for herbivores who eat plants exclusively–not even a termite can digest wood! Normally we are all dependent on our gut buddies to do the job of digesting this plant matter for us. (That big belly on a gorilla? It's a virtual fermentation vat filled with microbes breaking down the huge amount of plants it consumes!)

Cooking foods enabled humans to eat a more varied diet, as well as digest more nutrients. It also allowed us to eat certain foods that are inedible in raw form (yams and sweet potatoes, for instance), but which contain important nutrients. And the cooked starches from these tubers helped nourish our gut buddies. In this book, you'll learn how pressure cooking lectin-containing foods at very high heat has a similar effect—it enables you to extract more nutrients from foods, and eat some grains and legumes that are not only inedible raw, but are toxic unless cooked properly. Imagine where human evolution might be now if cavemen had had an Instant Pot!

The Seven Deadly Disruptors

In addition to the advent of agriculture, modern innovations to our lifestyle in the form of drugs, pesticides, and other chemicals have also had a deleterious effect on our health, and especially the health of our gut and gut buddies. If you've read *The Plant Paradox,* you'll know that I've identified seven specific toxins that are harming our health—I call them the "Seven Deadly Disruptors." I go into much more detail about these chemicals in my other books, but for our purposes here (and so we can get you cooking and improving your family's health faster!), I'll quickly summarize them.

1. BROAD-SPECTRUM ANTIBIOTICS. It must be said that these drugs can be a highly beneficial, life-saving treatment when used correctly. Unfortunately, today they are commonly overprescribed. Antibiotics are so effective that in addition to killing the pathogenic bad bugs, they also wipe out almost all of the trillions of friendly bacteria in your gut. And, bad news: your gut buddies don't grow back overnight if you swallow a probiotic or eat some yogurt. Think of a course of antibiotics like a forest fire. Even if you plant new seedlings after

the fire has wiped out all of the old trees, it takes a long time for a new forest to grow. But our exposure to antibiotics doesn't only come from swallowing a pill—every time we eat conventionally-raised beef and pork, or even farmed seafood, we're consuming the antibiotics given to those animals to keep them alive and fatten them up for slaughter. When you consume meat from these animals, your gut buddies take a hit.

2. NONSTEROIDAL ANTI-INFLAMMATORY DRUGS (NSAIDS). This class of drugs includes Ibuprofen (Motrin/Advil), naproxen (Aleve), Celebrex, and other pain relievers. NSAIDs damage the lining of your small intestine and colon, also targeted by lectins, and are a major and under-recognized cause of leaky gut. If these drugs are taken regularly, the result is more and more holes in the gut, which leads to increased inflammation, which means more pain—prompting you to take more NSAIDs. It's a terribly vicious cycle. The next time you reach for one of these pills or hand one to your child, ask yourself first if it is really necessary. Many times we take these drugs more out of comfort or habit than true need.

3. STOMACH ACID BLOCKERS. When we eat something (generally a food that contains lectins) that gives us indigestion or heartburn, we often reach for acid-blocking drugs like Zantac, Prilosec, Nexium, or Protonix to relieve our discomfort. These drugs, most of which are proton pump inhibitors (PPIs), reduce the production of stomach acid. That may seem like a good idea, except that stomach acid is what your body uses to neutralize harmful bacteria (aka, bad bugs) and partially digest lectins (they are proteins, after all; acid digests proteins). And the more bad bacteria you have, the less room and fewer resources your gut buddies have to thrive—which means your immune system takes a hit too. Is it any wonder that studies show that people who use acid blockers have three times the likelihood of getting pneumonia than those who do not? And don't get me started on the increased risk of dementia and heart failure while taking these drugs! Note: To any readers who have been diagnosed with Small Intestinal Bacteria Overgrowth (SIBO), please stop taking these drugs immediately, as they are especially harmful for you—the acid in your stomach prevents bad bugs, which meant to stay in your colon, from swimming upstream into you small bowel where they don't belong and can make you sick.

4. ARTIFICIAL SWEETENERS. I'm going to tell you something: I am still heartbroken about how damaging artificial sweeteners are. After all, I was a Diet Coke addict for years. I used to drink eight cans a day...and I was also seventy pounds

overweight. While these sweeteners are, indeed, calorie-free, they also decimate your gut buddies[2] while simultaneously triggering your brain to seek out more sweet flavors—prompting you to eat sugar in other forms.

5. ENDOCRINE DISRUPTORS. These chemicals, which are commonly found in plastics—including plastic wrap and food storage containers as well as personal care products (makeup, shampoo, soap, perfume, sunscreen, etc), household cleaners, carpeting, flame-retardant fabrics, and mattresses—have been shown to interfere with the normal functioning of your hormones. Exposure to them is linked to an array of health issues including diabetes, cancer, poor thyroid function, reproductive problems, and obesity.

In addition to plastics, beware of endocrine disruptors lurking in processed foods. Stabilizing agents such as butylated hydroxytoluene, or BHT, are used to extend the shelf life of whole grain products like breads and crackers. BHT can also be found in "healthy" industrially-raised chicken.

Sanitizer Makes You Sick

Antibacterial soaps and hand sanitizers have a great marketing gimmick going for them—they promise to kill every germ on your hands and protect you from getting sick. But the reality is, instead of keeping you healthy, those chemicals do the opposite: they decimate your microbiome and negatively impact your immune system, leaving you more exposed to illness. As a doctor, I know something about the importance of washing your hands. And my suggestion for keeping your family's hands clean? Good old-fashioned soap and water. There are lots of inexpensive, high-quality soaps out there—even better if you forgo the ones that come in a plastic dispenser and stick with bar soap. Dr. Bronner brand makes an excellent castile bar soap with a fresh, unobtrusive mint scent (derived from peppermint oil and not some nefarious chemical) and is fairly easy to find at Trader Joe's, Whole Foods, and a slew of other stores. Trust me, bar soap and water will do the trick!

6. GENETICALLY MODIFIED FOODS (GMOS) AND THE HERBICIDE ROUNDUP. Most genetically modified foods have been bred to withstand glyphosate, which is a key ingredient in the pesticide Roundup, made by Monsanto (now owned by Bayer, and Enlist, which is manufactured by Dow Chemical). Glyphosate has been classified as a "probable human carcinogen" by the World Health Organization. Amazingly, it is patented not as an herbicide, but as an antibiotic, meaning that it kills bacteria (including your gut microbes when you ingest it

in the food you eat). In rat studies, Roundup has also been found to contribute to fatty liver disease (an inflamed liver) even at low doses. When you consider that the liver is an organ that helps to filter out toxins from the body, it makes sense that exposure to Roundup would cause it to become inflamed.

Unlike non-GMO plants, many GMO plants have been engineered to survive when exposed to glyphosate. This means that farmers can drench their fields with the chemical to kill the weeds, while their main crop—typically corn, soy, or wheat—is unaffected. This is straightforward enough, and the takeaway is—don't buy GMO foods. Unfortunately, it's becoming a lot tougher for consumers to have transparency into how their food is produced, and some sneaky practices are at work. Farmers are using Roundup on non-GMO conventional crops as a desiccant to help accelerate crop death, because a dried-up plant is easier to harvest. Roundup is now being used on almost all conventionally-grown wheat, corn, oats, legumes, beans, and canola, which means it's more important than ever to select organic versions of these foods—as well as products that contain these ingredients, like breads, crackers, cereals, oatmeal, granola bars, and even wines and beers. In addition, glyphosate is present in the meat and dairy of animals who are fed non-organic grains.

7. BLUE LIGHT. Our bodies are finely tuned to react to the light we perceive via our optic nerve. When days are long and nights are short (in summer), we are cued to eat more and store fat to prepare us for the coming winter, when food was typically scarce. And when days are short and nights are long, our body gets a signal to burn stored fat since calories from food were generally reduced. These days, we spend most of our time staring at electronic devices that emit blue light—the part of the light spectrum that comprises daylight—prompting our internal clock to think it's summer all year long. Thus we are continually "preparing for winter," mistakenly consuming more calories and storing fat rather than burning it.

How Lectins Cause Weight Gain in You and Your Children

As you probably know from all of the press about gluten, wheat is an especially dense source of lectins. But in addition to gluten—which is actually not the worst offender among lectins—there is a particularly damaging lectin present in whole wheat foods called wheat germ agglutinin (WGA). WGA signals your body to store fat and has also been linked to celiac and heart diseases. But what is it about WGA that makes it so insidious? One of its sneaky qualities (which it shares with other lectins) is its ability to mimic insulin in the body.

Oh No, not those Os...!

Oats are a staple of many children's diets—from breakfast foods like oatmeal and cereal "O"s to oat bars and oatmeal cookies to the increasingly popular dairy alternative, oat milk. For generations, oats have been viewed as a "health food," and certainly a kid-friendly food. But oats are a lot less virtuous then you might think. For starters, most oats—even those advertised as "gluten-free"—contain a protein that cross-reacts with gluten, making them a hazard if anyone in your family has a gluten intolerance or allergy. In addition, oats do contain lectins (and are often contained in animal feed, which is already full of lectins from corn and soy).

But the most disturbing thing about oats is the way they are harvested. A recent study conducted by the international environmental group Friends of the Earth found that 100 percent of non-organic store-brand oat cereal samples tested positive for residues of glyphosate, the active ingredient in the herbicide Roundup. The average level of glyphosate detected in the samples was 360 parts per billion (ppb), which FOE noted is more than twice the level set by Environmental Working Group (EWG) scientists for lifetime cancer risk in children. This is because the common farming practice for conventionally-raised, non-GMO oats is to spray the crops with Roundup as a desiccant—to accelerate the drying process and make them easier to harvest. Because the herbicide is sprayed just before harvesting, you can bet that it is all over those dried oats and oat products you buy at the store. As noted on page 12, Roundup is a known neurotoxin and is not something you want to feed your children (or eat yourself!). I recommend avoiding all oats, but if you do choose to eat oats or oat products, please purchase only organic varieties!

A hormone made by your pancreas, insulin is released into your bloodstream in varying amounts in response to the amount of sugar and protein you eat. It helps to regulate your blood sugar levels by attaching to docks on fat, neuron, or muscle cells and ordering them to open up and let the glucose in. Once the glucose is moved into the cell, the insulin detaches, backs out of the dock, and all is well.

WGA acts similarly to insulin, but instead of docking only temporarily to a cell, it stays there indefinitely. Imagine being in a full parking lot and waiting for a space to open up—you circle and circle the lot, but no one ever comes back to move their car from a space. This is what happens when WGA parks in your cells—it causes sugar to circle through your blood stream, looking for a place to park. When it makes enough rounds, your body responds by telling the pancreas to produce more insulin so that the sugar can be escorted to a cell. But WGA keeps insulin out, too. Over time, this creates a dangerous cycle in which your body becomes less sensitive to the presence of insulin in the blood—a condition known as insulin resistance, or prediabetes.

WGA causes problems for all types of cells in the body. When it parks on the dock of a muscle cell, blocking sugar from entering, it starves your muscle of the energy it needs. Without glucose, your muscles can't retain their mass, let alone grow. If your muscle cells are continuously deprived of glucose, eventually some degree of muscle wasting will set in.

Just as WGA starves muscle cells, it also starves nerve cells, or neurons. Without adequate glucose, your brain can't function properly. In response to energy restriction, your poor hungry, fatigued brain sends an SOS signal in the form of hunger, prompting you to eat more calories—and you comply, often seeking those calories in the form of sugar and carbohydrates. Of course, you already have plenty of available calories, the brain just can't access them—so you end up consuming more energy than you need, leading to weight gain.

Finally, WGA also does a number on your fat cells. When WGA parks there it not only attaches, but also ushers in all the rejected sugar that's still circling the lot, which then gets stored as fat. So the sum result of WGA mimicking insulin is that your muscle cells shrink, your brain feels sluggish, your fat cells grow, and you find yourself overeating all the time. Does any of this sound vaguely familiar?

Bullied at School

Being a teenager is never easy—and it's even harder when you don't feel and look your best. Such was the case for 14-year-old Sophia. When she visited my office, she was suffering from terrible acne, and she was significantly overweight. She was miserable and told me that she was bullied at school. Blood tests revealed that she had very high insulin levels, high triglycerides, and all the markers for pre-diabetes and insulin resistance. Her vitamin D and Omega 3 levels were low, and her testosterone was elevated. This combination of symptoms often results in a diagnosis of Polycystic Ovarian Syndrome (PCOS).

I knew that the underlying problem was Sophia's diet. She was drinking soda and juice, eating cereal and processed foods, and overeating all of these foods because she never felt full. She was willing to give the Plant Paradox program a try, so we gave her and her mother the "Yes, Please" and "No, Thank You" food lists and scheduled a follow up visit.

Two months later, Sophia had lost 10 pounds; 6 months later she was down 20 pounds! Her skin had also improved remarkably. Sophia said the bullying has eased, but she wasn't satisfied. She would ask me, "Why can't I lose more weight faster, Dr. G?" I told her what I tell everyone: "Weight off fast will never last! Weight off slow, you're good to go!" Sophia is learning how to eat to support her health and she's learning how to break life-long habits—that takes time. But it is well worth the investment.

The last time I spoke with her mom, she told me that Sophia was happier, and more confident, than she'd ever seen her. And her PCOS symptoms? They've disappeared too.

Not All Lectins Are Bad

While a diet high in lectins spells trouble for your health, the reality is that as long as you're eating plants, lectins can't be completely avoided—and that's ok. In fact, in small amounts, they can actually be beneficial.

I know, I know: I've just explained in great detail that lectins are bad for you—how could they be good for you? The concept of "hormesis," which is used in the field of toxicology, can help us understand this seeming paradox. Hormesis shows us that sometimes substances that are toxic in large quantities are actually beneficial in smaller quantities. In other words, to borrow a turn of phrase from Paracelsus, the Renaissance physician known as the "father of toxicology:" "The dose makes the poison."

The takeaway? Eat a varied diet. One of my objectives with this book is to expand your repertoire to include all kinds of foods that your family may be missing out on. While it may initially seem that a lectin-limited eating plan is difficult to sustain, the reality is, there is a wide array of plants—like tubers, pressure-cooked beans, and leafy greens—that feed your gut buddies and provide your body with optimal nutrition.

So don't be afraid of plants—most of them are more friend than foe. And don't worry if you've been eating a lot of the ones that fall into the "foe" category: It's never too late to reverse the damage done by lectins! No matter your current state of wellbeing, you have the power to turn things around. As I've described in my previous books, I've witnessed incredible transformations in my patients' health when they change their diets. Many have reversed chronic illnesses such as heart disease, type 2 diabetes, and autoimmune diseases. Others have healed longstanding digestive woes, lost weight, cleared brain fog, and regained their sense of vitality.

Of course, the Plant Paradox program is designed not only to help reverse these conditions and symptoms, but also to prevent them from occurring. That's why your committment to improving your family's health is so important. You can give your children every advantage they need and deserve to live a long and happy life—just by changing the food you pack in their lunch boxes every day.

On that note, let's take a closer look at what exactly is in those lunch boxes.

chapter two

Separating Fact from Fiction in Kids' Nutrition

After countless conversations with patients and friends who ask me about the best way to feed their families, it's become clear to me that there's a lot of confusion out there when it comes to nutrition not only for adults but for kids as well.

If you're reading this book and you're a parent, you're probably already an avid consumer of health information, and you're eager to do anything and everything you can to give your child or children the best possible start in life. For that, I applaud you: because truly, nothing sets up a child for long-term health, vitality, and proper development as much as the nutrition they eat. Especially from newborn to age three, when little bodies are just forming—food affects everything from the makeup of their microbiome to the strength of their immune system to the development of their brain.

That said, it is never too late to make a meaningful impact on your children's health. Whether your kids are toddlers, grade schoolers, middle schoolers, or even practically adults, not only will the food you serve them affect their wellbeing, but the way you eat at home—preparing healthy foods together, eating family dinners, valuing high-quality ingredients—will set a powerful example that your kids will take with them long after they've left the house.

My goal is to empower you to feed your family the kind of food that will not only make everyone healthier and happier, but also give you the tools to make this healthy eating simple and sustainable. With that in mind, let's set the record straight once and for all and separate fact from fiction when it comes to kids' nutrition.

The Lunchbox Diaries

To my mind, nothing quite sums up the misinformation about how we feed our kids more than the all-American lunchbox: A peanut butter and jelly sandwich, made with squishy processed bread, served with a side of milk, and perhaps some fruit—an apple, a bunch of grapes, a box of raisins. Even if that sandwich is made with whole-grain bread; even if the peanut butter is "organic;" even if the milk is "skim milk," this is still far from a healthy lunch. In fact it might as well be dynamite for your kids' gut buddies.

Yet many well-intentioned parents are fooled into believing that such a meal provides their children with the fuel they need to grow and learn.

It's not your fault. When you go to the grocery store, watch television, or read advice in health magazines or online, you are bombarded with conflicting information. Unfortunately, for the most part, what you're being told (or rather sold) is either processed food or purported "health food" that's anything but healthy.

It's easy enough to isolate the processed stuff: if it comes in a box, if the nutrition label features a list of hard-to-pronounce ingredients, or if the food has undergone a "process" to arrive at its final state—then it's processed. But harder to identify are the foods you've long believed are healthy: whole grains, milk, and fruit, to name a few from our lunch example. For those of you who have already experienced the benefits of the Plant Paradox plan, the information I'm about to share won't be surprising. But what I want all of my readers to understand is that the Plant Paradox plan's benefits are not limited to adults. Children who eat the foods on this protocol are not deficient in any nutrients, and they're not deprived or suffering from missing anything in their diets. Rather, they thrive on this program and learn how to make healthy foods choices from a young age, which is a skill that will last a lifetime.

The Plant Paradox program requires a multifaceted approach to lifestyle change, but once you get the hang of it, not only will it empower you to give your family the best nutrition possible, it will also, believe it or not, *save* you time in the kitchen and money at the grocery store. And that sounds pretty good, doesn't it? Now, I won't sugarcoat this: it will require some investment of time up front, including planning your meals each week. But getting organized is essential to making any big change stick. You will use your menu plan as a map for your weekly grocery shopping, too. In some cases, one parent may be able to swing by the store (instead of the drive-thru or pizza place) on their way home from work and grab an ingredient or two. In other cases, you may be able to only squeeze in a weekly grocery trip, which will require you to plan a little more thoughtfully. You'll also do some batch cooking and prepping over the weekend, so it's easier to make dinners (and pack lunches) on school nights.

Now, let's get to the issue at hand: how to feed your family. I know that what I'm about to share is unsettling, but the information you're getting from trusted sources, including the government, and often your pediatrician, is flawed. Nothing against your pediatrician—remember, I've worked in pediatrics myself—but most doctors aren't given nutrition classes in medical school. The advice they offer their patients is typically based not on the latest research, but on the USDA food pyramid. And let's be clear about one thing: the U.S. Department of Agriculture's job is to sell agricultural products. What does the U.S. produce in mass quantities? Corn, wheat, soybeans, cow's milk, beef, pork, and chicken. Is it any wonder the USDA's guidelines are predicated on consuming these products?

So let's take a closer look at that pyramid, and what the USDA suggests you feed your family.

US DEPARTMENT OF AGRICULTURE FOOD PYRAMID

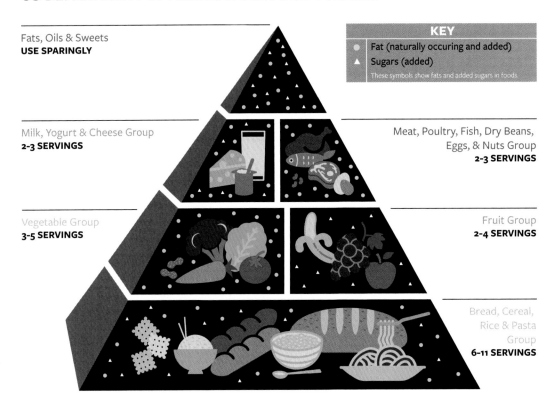

Fats, Oils & Sweets
USE SPARINGLY

KEY
Fat (naturally occuring and added)
Sugars (added)
These symbols show fats and added sugars in foods.

Milk, Yogurt & Cheese Group
2-3 SERVINGS

Meat, Poultry, Fish, Dry Beans,
Eggs, & Nuts Group
2-3 SERVINGS

Vegetable Group
3-5 SERVINGS

Fruit Group
2-4 SERVINGS

Bread, Cereal,
Rice & Pasta
Group
6-11 SERVINGS

As you can see, the base of the pyramid is comprised of grains such as bread, pasta, rice, and cereal—all lectin-loaded, processed foods. Above grains we have 3 to 5 servings of vegetables (great!) and 2 to 4 servings of fruit—a quantity that, as we will discuss shortly, is hugely excessive. What's above fruit and veggies? Why 2 to 3 servings of good old-fashioned dairy products of course—as well as 2 to 3 *daily* servings of meat. At the top? Fats, oils, and sweets to be consumed "sparingly." This may be the sole place I am in agreement with the USDA—sweets should be consumed exceedingly sparingly. But healthy fats and oils? Let's just say, they are a lot better for your child's growing brain than a bowl of Wheaties.

It's time to take a closer look at what we're feeding our kids. To kick things off, I've identified the top five "healthy" foods that parents are encouraged to feed their kids, because I want to explore the reasons why they aren't actually so healthy. There's a very good chance you may have several of these items in your kitchen now, but after reading this, I doubt they'll be in your home for long!

The 5 Fictitious Foods (That Are Not Healthy for Kids!)

1. COW'S MILK

Milk is on the high honor roll of healthy foods for kids. Parents are advised to begin giving their children whole milk the moment they are weaned from breast milk or formula—as early as age one. And remember those milk mustache ads and the campaign to get kids to drink more milk to build healthy bones and teeth? We have long been marketed the idea that milk is a food that "does a body good." I beg to differ.

Nearly all of cow's milk in the U.S. and Canada comes from breeds of cows (including the most common breed worldwide, the Holstein) that produce a lectin-like protein known as casein A1, which is converted in your body to the protein beta-casomorphin (BCM), an opiod-like substance that may explain why milk is so addicting and helps adults and children feel comforted. Unfortunately, this protein also attaches to the pancreas's insulin-producing cells, known as beta cells, which prompts an immune attack on the pancreas.

Research indicates this protein may be a primary cause of type 1 diabetes.[3] BCM also stimulates inflammation. If you suspect you or your child are "lactose-intolerant," it's likely that you're actually experiencing the discomfort of this inflammatory response, not a problem with lactose.

Many times, parents of infants and toddlers struggle to accept the idea that they don't need to give their children milk to ensure healthy growth and development. I understand their dilemma—just about every authority new parents rely on for accurate information suggests just the opposite of what I'm saying. To help assuage their fears, I explain why milk is in no way essential for their child's wellbeing.

First, it's important to understand that all cow's milk is not only dense in calories, but is loaded with insulin-like growth factor (IGF-1), which, as the name implies, prompts rapid growth and weight gain. This is a benefit for calves: size is a valuable asset in the animal world. Bigger animals are more likely to survive and are less likely to be attacked by a predator. Amazingly, however, your child is not a calf that needs to grow rapidly! Quite the opposite: humans are designed to grow slowly; that's why human breastmilk has much less IGF-1 than cow's milk. As long as your child is eating a varied diet that includes plenty of calcium-rich foods like spinach, sweet potatoes, figs (they can be reconstituted in warm water), and pressure-cooked beans or lentils—all pureed, if necessary—he or she *will not be stunted or deficient in any key nutrients*. And if you never introduce milk in the first place, your child will never miss it.

If your family is currently consuming conventional cow's milk and/or cow's milk yogurt, cottage cheese, most cheeses, and ice cream, I recommend removing these products from your and their diet. Luckily, due the popularity of the vegan and vegetarian lifestyles, there many widely available and delicious substitutes for these foods, including goat, sheep, and coconut milks, cheese, and yogurts (be sure to avoid those with added sugars) and pili nut yogurt (sold under the brand name Lavva). Your kids can still enjoy ice cream as well—there is a wide variety of coconut milk–based options available (again, avoid those high in sugar), just be sure to steer clear of soy-based dairy alternatives, as these products are typically made with GMO soy and are high in lectins. Of course, the best way to give your kids healthy ice cream treats is to make them at home, where you can control every ingredient—such as the Keto Kids' Fudge Pops (page 210) and Almond Butter and Jelly Popsicles (page 213), which are simple to make and a huge hit with kids!

Vitamin D

The one beneficial thing about cow's milk for growing kids? In this country, milk is fortified with vitamin D, which is essential for young, growing bones to develop properly. Studies have also shown that higher levels of vitamin D in childhood translates to lower cholesterol levels in kids.[4] Unfortunately, most adults and children are deficient in vitamin D. Our body needs exposure to sunlight to convert vitamin D to its usable form, and as more and more kids spend their free time looking at screens rather than outside playing in the sunshine, pediatricians are seeing more and more vitamin D deficiencies in their young patients.

The American Academy of Pediatrics recommends a minimum of 600 IUs daily of vitamin D for children ages 1 to 7, and 800 IUs daily for children ages 8 and older. I disagree. Almost all children I see with allergies, asthma, eczema, or other autoimmune diseases, have very low vitamin D levels. Kids above age 7or 8 can easily take 2,000 IUs a day of vitamin D3. I have yet to see a single case of vitamin D toxicity in my thousands of patients who take vitamin D supplements.

In addition to supplementation with pills or gummies, be sure to give your kids plenty of vitamin D–rich foods like egg yolks and salmon. And encourage them to play outside in the sun!

2. WHOLE GRAINS

Chances are, for most of your life you've believed that whole grains are a healthy choice, and you've gone out of your way, and spent extra money, to make sure your family eats whole wheat, multi-grain, seeded everything. You buy the brown bread with lots of texture; you make oatmeal for breakfast; you serve quinoa at dinner; you order brown rice with your sushi. You want to feed your family right.

I'm truly sorry to tell you this, but it's all a myth. Whole grains are far from a health food. Yes, they are slower-digesting than processed grains that have had the hull and germ removed. But it's those components—the hull of the seed—that contain the greatest concentration of lectins. Whole grains are highly inflammatory, even more so than their de-hulled counterparts like white bread and white rice.

Whole grains are also carbohydrates that convert to sugar in the body, which means they are a source of unnecessary pounds as well. In addition to promoting weight gain, wheat triggers an opiate-like response in your brain, which prompts you to crave more and more. For many, including kids, these carbohydrates also cause brain fog and fatigue.

So where does our belief in the "goodness" of whole grains originate? It all started with Will Keith Kellogg, founder of Kellogg's brand. Around the turn of the twentieth century, Kellogg and his brother, John Harvey Kellogg, devised a way to process corn into crunchy flakes, which they recommended for their ability to help keep people "regular." This was the beginning of massive advertising push—and a fiction—that persists to this day: that cereal, and whole grains, are the cornerstone of a healthy breakfast. Top it off with a little cow's milk, and you have a prototypical kid's breakfast—one that is brimming with inflammatory, gut-punishing lectins.

I am not going to suggest that your child skips breakfast (though it's certainly beneficial for adults to do so on occasion), but I do suggest your children eat a low-carb, keto-friendly breakfast that will keep their blood sugar stable and provide them with filling, nutrient-dense fuel for the day. In other words, put down that box of "healthy" cereal or that packet of instant oatmeal, which carries little to no nutritional value, and make your kids an omelet instead. No time to cook in the morning? Hard boil some eggs in advance and create breakfast bowls with a hard-boiled egg and half an avocado sprinkled with sea salt and drizzled with olive oil. With that combination of healthy fats and protein, their little minds and bodies will be well-prepared for the school day ahead!

3. FRUIT

Another fact that many parents find shocking is that fruit should be enjoyed in moderation—yes, even for children. I realize this one is particularly tough because fruit is such an easy and convenient snack. Who hasn't told their kid to grab an apple when they complain of being hungry? Of course, an apple is still better than a bag of chips or some other type of processed food, but it's not the best choice.

Incidentally, as with cereal, there is an interesting story behind our embrace of fruit—in particular, bananas. The idea that fruit was an essential part of a healthy diet originated in an advertising campaign devised by the United Fruit Company (Chiquita Bananas), which claimed that bananas cured celiac disease and offered a coupon for a free bunch of bananas in— you guessed it!—Kellogg's Corn Flakes boxes. United Fruit Company even paid doctors to promote bananas for kids' health!

So, why do I suggest limiting fruit? Mostly because it is loaded with sugar—even more so today, as modern fruit has been hybridized for high sugar content. (Ever wonder why the Honey Crisp apple is so popular? It's been bred to taste extra sweet!) And yes, it is "natural" sugar, but fructose, the sugar found in fruit, inflicts serious damage on your liver and kidneys. A recent study out of UCLA showed that a diet high in fructose can lead to insulin resistance, which in turn slows the brain and impairs memory and learning.[5]

As you can see on page 20, the USDA recommends eating 2 to 4 servings of fruit a day for adults, and their recommendation for children is virtually the same. That's more than twice the amount of fruit you and your children should be eating! I want you to start thinking of fruit as nutritious candy. While fruit does contain beneficial vitamins, minerals, fiber, antioxidants, and polyphenols, you need only a small serving to get the benefits. I'm not suggesting that you have to eradicate fruit from your and your kids' diets—just make some modifications to how much and which fruits they eat.

FRUIT GUIDELINES

- Offer your kids in-season fruits; always choose organic, and try to buy from local farmers.

- Change up your family's on-the-go snacks to options that provide protein and fat instead of carbs and sugar: try offering a handful of macadamia nuts, pistachios, or walnuts; unsweetened almond butter with celery sticks; or a small container of coconut, goat's, pili nut, or sheep's milk yogurt.

- Aim for lower-sugar, high-nutrient fruits like berries, pomegranate seeds, and citrus fruits.

- Avoid most tropical fruits (with the exceptions below), which are especially high in sugar.

- Feel free to eat the following tropical fruits year-round in their unripe form: bananas, mangoes, and papayas.

- Make fruit a treat and serve no more than once a day. To make it a dessert-like indulgence, try topping fruits like berries, plums, or nectarines with a little bit of whipped coconut cream.

Yes, Sugar Is As Bad As You Think It Is.

I don't have to tell you that sugar is terrible for you, and your kids. Not only do sugary foods have no place on the Plant Paradox program, they should have no place in anyone's diet. But despite the fact that we know sugar is hazardous to our health, many of us keep eating it. And thanks to peer pressure, social customs, and sheer convenience, so do our kids. Many parents feel pressure to "let their kids enjoy childhood" by giving into pleas for sweets, from candy and cookies to juice and soda. And seemingly-healthy kid's foods—including yogurts, granola, cereals, and energy bars—even contain crazy amounts of hidden sugars. (Not that you're buying your kids any of these processed foods, right?)

Shockingly, as much as 40 percent of American healthcare dollars are spent to treat diseases directly related to the overconsumption of sugar—that's more than $1 trillion invested annually in treating sugar and junk-food related ailments.[4] Numerous studies have shown that excess sugar intake from processed foods may negatively impact your children's cognition. Soda and fruit juice consumption can raise a child's risk of obesity by 60 percent per daily serving.[5] And as we know, obesity is a risk factor for type 2 diabetes.[6]

So, to the parents who tell me they feel guilty for denying their children the simple pleasures of childhood, I say: you are not denying them a thing—you are giving them the precious gift of health. One day they will thank you!

- Limit serving sizes of fruit to about a half a cup (taking into consideration age and type of fruit).

- Avoid fruit juices of all types—even those that are "fresh squeezed." This is merely mainlining sugar!

There is one exception to the fruit rule: avocadoes! Technically a fruit, the humble avocado is one of the healthiest foods you can eat, and you and your kids should feel free to enjoy them year-round.

4. PEANUTS AND PEANUT BUTTER

The peanut, which originated in the Americas and was introduced to Europe by Christopher Columbus, is the most popular nut in the U.S. And guess what? It's not even a nut! It's a legume and it is loaded with lectins.

You might be wondering about peanut allergies—these days it seems like more kids are allergic to peanuts than ever before. And in fact they are. All food allergies, including peanut allergies, are on the rise. As you may already know, peanut allergies are so dangerous and widespread, many school lunchrooms are now equipped with EpiPens, and some school campuses have gone peanut-free. While the ubiquity and severity of these allergies is a somewhat modern phenomenon, the reality is that 94 percent of humans carry an antibody to the peanut lectin.[6] Most people have some sensitivity to peanuts, and humans have no business eating peanuts or peanut products.

Peanuts and peanut butter tend to be thought of as kids' foods, so you'll find them in just about every packaged food marketed to kids (and parents)—from trail mixes to granola bars to cereals to "healthy" cookies. Here's the good news: as long as you're avoiding packaged foods, you can avoid a lot of peanuts too! A win-win. And organic almond butter is a great swap for peanut butter—use it in everything from sandwiches to baked goods—your kids may love the flavor even more than their beloved peanut butter!

To Dose or Not to Dose?

Due to the surge in peanut allergies, many pediatricians now advise parents to begin introducing small amounts of peanut butter to babies as young as six months old. The thinking here is that earlier exposure means a reduced risk of allergies as the child grows, with the small doses functioning much like a vaccine to "educate" the immune system not to react to peanuts. I understand that this may seem like a logical intervention to ensure your child's safety, but as you might expect, I disagree with the idea of introducing peanuts in any form.

Instead of relying on peanut butter to educate a child's immune system, a better bet is to rely on a healthy microbiome. Gut bugs "talk" to the immune system and teach it what is a threat and what isn't. For babies, building a healthy microbiome means avoiding exposure to endocrine-disrupting chemicals (see pages 12–13 for more details), breastfeeding when possible[7], and avoiding unnecessary cycles of antibiotics. For older children, it means feeding them a varied diet of gut-supporting foods and avoiding lectins (as well as endocrine disruptors and antibiotics, unless essential). The best defense against life-changing allergies isn't a good offense—it's a good gut!

5. BEANS AND LENTILS

Many pediatricians will advise you to introduce these forms of plant-based protein as "first foods"—infants throughout America are fed mushy beans and lentils by well-intentioned parents who think they are giving their little ones the building blocks of life. Unfortunately, like peanuts, beans and lentils are legumes and are, therefore, rich in lectins. But it's not all doom and gloom: you can still safely feed these foods to your children, as long as you are conscientious how you source and prepare them. Always look for organic beans and lentils, as many are GMO crops and/or grown with pesticides. And be sure to soak your beans overnight before cooking them in the pressure-cooker, which helps to remove the lectins during the cooking process.

For an easy shortcut, look for Eden Foods organic canned beans, which are soaked and then pressure-cooked in the cans. Just rinse and serve!

The State of (Student) Union

If you're reading this book, chances are you're already aware of some sobering statistics about the state of children's health in this country. Between 1970 and 2009, daily caloric intake for kids rose by about 425 calories on average—a 20 percent increase—largely driven by increased sugar and processed food consumption, and constant advertising of junk food to children.[8]

Not only have the variety of temptations increased, so too have portion sizes. In a study that examined what Americans ate over the 30-year period from 1986 to 2016, researchers found that the total number of entrees, desserts, and sides increased by 226 percent, or 22.9 percent per year of the study. What's more, the calories in all three categories increased significantly as well, with the largest increase being desserts, followed by entrees. Worse yet, a study that looked at kids' ability to portion control found that children's caloric intake increased with a larger portion size. In other words, it's up to you to help your children to determine what constitutes a healthy amount of food.[9]

Increasingly, our diets have become filled with processed vegetable oils, which are high in a type of fat called omega-6 that is linked to disease and inflammation. These fats are also present in grain-fed meat, dairy, and eggs, whereas beneficial omega-3 fats are found in the oils of fish, particularly wild-caught fatty fish (farmed fish contain a significantly lower amount of these healthful fats).[10] Soybean oil, which is loaded with lectins, is the most commonly-consumed fat in the U.S. and plays a significant role in the development of obesity and diabetes.[11]

Today, nearly 20 percent of American children and nearly 40 percent of adults are obese. And as obesity rates rise, so do related-health problems, including increased risks of type 2 diabetes and cancer. Obesity in youth can also trigger earlier puberty in both boys and girls. One study that tracked hormonal changes in boys ages 4 to 7 determined that those who were obese had greater odds of starting puberty before the age of 9.[12] While this has been previously observed in girls, the fact that obesity also affects the maturation of boys further cements concerns about the wide-ranging effects of obesity in children.

While much of childhood obesity can be attributed to eating a diet high in junk food and processed food, the 7 Deadly Disruptors play a role as well. Household products such as hand sanitizers, antibacterial soaps, nonstick cookware, plastic wrap, and more expose you and your children to hormone-disrupting toxins that both interfere with the normal functioning of your endocrine system and cause the body to store fat.[13]

So, what can we do to start turning the tide on our health and our family's health? The answer is really very simple: cook and eat at home more often. Make family meals vegetable-centric, with a good portion of healthy fats, some protein, and limited portions of in-season fruit, preferably all organic. Real food is, at its core, straightforward. It's not a bunch of hard-to-pronounce ingredients and chemicals. Think about it—if chemicals are added to a food to preserve it and destroy bacteria, guess what they're doing to your gut buddies? That's right, they take a hit too. Consumption of processed foods has even been linked to an increased risk of cancer and early death.[14] By cutting out or reducing processed and high-carb food at home, you are reducing your whole family's risk of obesity and chronic diseases, as well as tooth decay[15] (and oral health is critical to overall health).

When you get the junk foods out your house, you will notice a huge difference in your family's health—and fast. As inspiration to make these changes, let me share with you the results of a famous study on kid's nutrition. Years ago, a school in Appleton, Wisconsin, changed its school food program, eliminating extra sugars and processed food and instead preparing healthy, organic meals for breakfast and lunch at school. Administrators also engaged with parents about how to make healthy dinner choices at home. The results of the study were astounding. Test scores and student behavior improved, truancy rates dropped dramatically, and kids complained of fewer health-related problems. Teachers also reported enhanced concentration skills in their pupils. One teacher even said that she saw these changes begin to take place "overnight."[16] If that's not motivation to start changing the way your family eats, I don't know what is!

After removing processed carbs, sugar, and all other junk food from your home, I recommend increasing your family's consumption of foods rich in omega-3 fats. These are foods like wild-caught salmon, flaxseeds, and walnuts. At the same time, you want to decrease consumption of omega-6 rich foods (think deep-fried foods cooked in lectin-rich, highly processed oils such as canola, soy, and peanut), which are highly inflammatory. It's important to keep in mind though, that simply cutting down on omega-6 fats and eating a few more servings of omega-3s a week isn't enough. EPA and DPA, two long-chain omega-3 acids, are critical for brain and heart health[17], and most people aren't getting enough of these nutrients. In fact, a recent study showed that children and adults who made changes to their diet to minimize omega-6 fats and increase consumption of omega-3s still didn't consume enough EPA or DHA.

The standard American diet has long been criticized for its low EPA and DHA content, and even health-conscious adults are challenged to meet their needs given the lack of access (and also prohibitive costs) of some of the best sources of the longer chain omega-3: wild-caught fatty fish and shellfish, and grass-fed-and-finished beef.[18] But it is well worth the extra effort and money to consume these fats, whether through food or supplementation. Many diseases such as ADHD, depression, cardiovascular disease, and metabolic syndrome (to name a few) could be improved by increasing omega-3 consumption.[19] In addition, higher DHA intake in children has been shown to correlate with improved school performance!

Let me sum up with this fact: When that Wisconsin school experimented with adding "junk food days" to their new, healthy food program, guess what happened? In the days following these indulgences, students complained of stomach aches, feelings of sadness, and lethargy.[20] It's worth it to make these changes for your family. So let's take a look at some strategies to make the transition to a Plant Paradox lifestyle a little easier on you and your kids.

Getting Your Family on Board with The Plant Paradox: A Cheat Sheet

1. CHOOSE ONE FOOD/ONE MEAL AT A TIME. Don't try to change everything overnight. Not only is it difficult to do a 180 on a practical level, but such an abrupt transition is difficult for the whole family on an emotional and psychological

level. Bring your kids into the process and give them some control. For instance, if you want to take the strategy of cutting out one food a day, maybe let your kids vote on which foods are the first to go.

2. **PLAN AHEAD.** I can't stress this enough: Being organized and planning your meals is the best way to ensure success. Make sure to keep some go-to foods on hand: Omega-3 or pastured eggs, frozen vegetables, coconut milk, avocadoes. Prep vegetables for snacks and meals and wash, dry, and properly store your leafy greens. Buy a salad spinner, and let your kids "run" it. Stock a few basic components, like cauliflower rice, miracle noodles, and Quorn or tempeh, that can be easily thrown together for dinner, preventing you from having any excuses on a busy weeknight.

3. **COOK IN LARGE BATCHES.** Double or triple the recipe you're making, and freeze leftovers for those days when you don't have time to cook. Even better if you can pre-portion into individual servings before freezing. Or save leftovers in the fridge for quick lunches during the week.

4. **GET YOUR KIDS IN THE KITCHEN.** Involving your kids in the preparation of meals—even if they're just stirring the ingredients—will help them feel more invested in the meal and more interested in what's on their plates. And having some little helpers in the kitchen cuts down on your prep time. Both of my grandchildren love to cook with their parents (particularly when it comes to making cookies and pancakes)!

5. **OFFER CHOICES.** Give your children choices when it comes to their meals. Let them reject one vegetable on their plate. (I had to hide my peas growing up! Little did I know I was rejecting lectin-rich legumes at a tender age.) As long as they are eating a variety of healthy foods, it's okay for kids to abstain from the things they truly cannot stomach. It's important to keep mealtimes as stress-free as possible so that kids don't develop negative or anxious feelings about food. Remember, their taste buds are still evolving! And no, when they reject a food on their plate, don't you have to give them what they want instead. They will not starve. I guarantee it.

6. **HYDRATE WISELY.** Serve water at mealtimes and in between meals. Cut out juice and soda completely, even the low carb or sugar free versions. Same goes for sports drinks and sugary or artificially-sweetened iced teas and lemonades. Once your family's taste buds adjust, you'll find they actually start craving water and choosing it to quench their thirst.

7. **EMBRACE YOUR PRESSURE COOKER AND/OR SLOW COOKER.** Let these two gadgets make your life in the kitchen easier. Part 2 of this book is loaded with new and easy recipes for using these appliances. With a slow cooker, you can just throw together a few ingredients in the morning and then enjoy a meal when you come home after work, without the stress of trying to pull together a meal at the last second when you and the whole family are hungry, tried, or even worse, "hangry." No time in the morning? No worries! An Instant Pot or other electric pressure cooker may be the ultimate "fast food" miracle. And remember, make a double batch and freeze the leftovers.

8. **SNACK SMART.** Stock your fridge and pantry with healthy snacks. If there are delicious, healthy options available, you and your family won't miss the processed stuff you used to munch on.

What to Expect When You're Expecting (or Expecting to Expect)

If you don't have a family now but are planning to start one soon—or if you are already expecting—then I don't need to tell you that prenatal nutrition is of the utmost importance for the health of both mother and baby. I get a lot of questions from patients and readers about the best way to eat during pregnancy, so I wanted to take a pause here to touch on my recommendations (if this doesn't apply to you, feel free to turn to Chapter 3!).

Before we go further, I want to say that good nutrition isn't only about the growing baby—it's also about the mother! Too often we speak to expecting mothers as though they are little more than incubators, offering advice solely under the guise of "what is good for the baby." I want to be clear that it is just as important for expecting and new mothers to care for themselves, to nourish themselves with healthy foods, and to keep their stress levels to a minimum by not overthinking every small choice. As long as they are eating well the majority of the time, their baby will be just fine.

With that said, the nutrients that fuel a fetus's development are also beneficial for mothers. So, what are those nutrients, and when do you need them? Well, the answer is, earlier than you might think. Obstetricians recommend women start taking a prenatal vitamin (not a general multivitamin) six months before planning to conceive,[21] and I agree that this is the right window for making nutritional changes to support a healthy pregnancy. Prenatal vitamins help to ensure a woman's body has the nutrients it needs to support new life, and recently they have also been shown to have a protective effect against autism. A study out of the University of California, Davis, concluded that mothers who took prenatal vitamins during their first month of pregnancy reduced their child's risk of autism by more than half.[22]

I also recommend supplementing with the active forms of B12 and Folate in the forms of Methyl B12 and methylfolate, to help protect against common genetic disorders. Another source of protective compounds can be found right in the produce aisle, in the form of pomegranates, which are one of the most polyphenol-rich foods in the world. (You can also buy pomegranate extract, which is sugar-free.) Polyphenols are "eaten" by gut buddies that convert them into compounds which help protect a developing child's brain[23] and heart, and may even help train the immune system.

Many obstetricians will also advise women to take omega-3 and DHA supplements, which support healthy brain development in the fetus. As you know, the American diet is sorely lacking in EPA and DHA, and there is no doubt that DHA is essential for healthy brain development. In fact, so important is DHA that a baby will "steal" (borrow?) almost 90 percent of its mother's DHA to build its own brain! I recommend all pregnant women, or women who are planning a pregnancy, take about 1,000 mg of fish oil or algae-derived DHA per day.

Eating for Two

I had just finished giving a lecture on the Plant Paradox at a seminar when a man approached me wondering if he could ask a few more questions. He explained that he was looking for information to help his wife, who suffered from rheumatoid arthritis (RA). She took immunosuppressant drugs, which clearly helped her manage her symptoms, but despite the fact that the couple had been trying to conceive for several years, she had not been able to get pregnant. Moreover, they were both afraid of the unknown effects the drugs she was taking might have on a baby if she were to become pregnant.

I offered to help and ran his wife's bloodwork, which revealed the classic markers for RA were positive, despite being on medication, and, she had very low levels of vitamin D and omega-3s. We began supplementation and started the Plant Paradox protocol. Three months later, her markers for RA were negative, and her vitamin D levels improved as well. We stopped her immunosuppressant drugs and gave her pre- and probiotics daily. Repeat blood work showed no recurrence of RA markers.

Shortly thereafter I got the call I had been hoping for: they were expecting! During the wife's pregnancy I prescribed increasing her fish oil supplementation and made sure she took methyl B12 and methyl folate. She continued to follow the Plant Paradox program. Today the couple has welcomed a healthy baby boy, and Mom has remained free from painful RA symptoms.

In addition to taking a supplemental DHA, one of the best ways to get the recommended amount of DHA is to consume on a weekly basis 8 to 12 ounces of oily fish, like wild-caught mackerel, sardines, and wild salmon, but with the cost of wild fish and possible contamination with mercury, I prefer getting your DHA from supplements. I also encourage pregnant women to keep in mind that a high intake of omega-6 fatty acids (found in processed food, fast foods, and vegetable oils) during pregnancy has been shown to predispose babies to obesity both in childhood and later in life, which lays the groundwork for numerous health problems down the road.[24] And researchers who performed a statistical analysis found that a higher omega-6 to omega-3 ratio during a mother's pregnancy was associated with a higher risk her child developing symptoms of ADHD around seven years of age.[25]

Another consideration for pregnant women is to avoid excess sugar, particularly processed sugar. Sugar negatively impacts cognition for babies in utero,[26] and one study found that drinking sugar-sweetened beverages in particular increases the risk of harm to the fetus's brain. "Diet" drinks didn't fare any better—they too were found to adversely impact child cognition.[27] I encourage all expecting moms to drink plenty of water or unsweetened tea (especially green tea, for its polyphenol content) as their beverage of choice—their growing bodies absolutely need hydration to support the function of two people!

The Importance of Choosing Organic

We all know how important it is to choose organic foods whenever possible, and eating organic is doubly important for pregnant women. But what you might not know is that new research points to the importance of eating organic foods even when couples are trying to conceive. A study published in the *Journal of the American Medical Association* found that pesticides can affect fertility in both women and men.[28] For men in particular, pesticides can alter DNA, causing gene mutations that may result in birth defects, or an outright inability to conceive.[29] And it goes without saying that this is a time to avoid exposure to the endocrine-disrupting chemicals listed on page 12, which can cause hormonal problems that have been shown to negatively impact fertility.[30]

I also get a lot of questions from new moms about how best to feed their babies, and whether breastfeeding is essential. New motherhood is challenging enough, so instead of adopting the mantra "breast is best," I like to support the idea that "fed is best." If your baby is healthy, growing, and thriving—you can hardly wish for more!

When it comes to formula, my advice is to look for varieties that contain pre- and post-biotics, DHA, B12, and folate, to make sure the baby is getting all of his or her nutritional needs met. If a new mother chooses to and is able to breastfeed, her diet postpartum continues to be just as critical to her baby's health as it was when she was planning and expecting her baby. I recommend continued supplementation with prenatal vitamins and DHA (1,000 mg), as these nutrients will be passed onto babies in breast milk.[31] And remember my famous saying: You are what you eat, but you are what the thing you are eating, ate. The same goes for babies—they literally eat what their mothers eat! Finally, I cannot stress enough the recommendation for breastfeeding moms to take a high-quality probiotic daily and feed their gut bugs with prebiotic foods like yams, jicama, Belgium endive and Sunchokes to name a few. The health of the baby's microbiome is a direct reflection of its mother's microbiome.

For all new moms, nutrition is an essential component of the postpartum recovery and healing process. Women not only lose blood (and therefore, iron) during birth, they also "lose" (or, donate) a lot of vitamins and DHA as they grow their babies. I encourage all new moms to increase their consumption of dark green leafy vegetables like spinach, which are iron rich, and take a vitamin C supplement twice a day near meals to help their bodies absorb that iron. Increasing your healthy fat intake from sources like avocadoes and olive oil is important too, and offers the side benefit of helping the body more easily shed the weight of pregnancy. And even for moms who aren't breastfeeding, I still recommend taking a DHA supplement—at least 1,000 mg. I've seen a number of new mothers suffering from postpartum depression, and when I run their bloodwork, it turns out that they have very low levels of DHA. Supplementation of this critical fatty acid really makes a big difference in their recovery.

Alright: Now you that you are armed with the facts (minus the fiction) about kids' nutrition, it's time to dive into the Plant Paradox program and make it a family affair. Are you ready? Let's go!

Breastmilk and the Microbiome

Breast milk is a treasure trove of nutrition for babies in many ways, and one is that is helps to set up a healthy microbiome for life. Recent research has shown that yeasts, other fungi, and bacteria in breast milk provide crucial microorganisms to the infant's developing gut biome. The presence of fungal cells within the breast milk also suggests that breast milk could influence the development of infants' mycobiota, a newly discovered component of our overall holobiome, which is made up of (beneficial) fungi.[32]

In addition, oligosaccharides, the naturally occurring sugars in mother's milk, serve as food for the baby's gut buddies and help to shape his or her microbiome and boost immunity. Breast milk is so beneficial to an infant's immune system that exclusively breastfed babies have been found to have lower infant mortality rates from common childhood illnesses such as diarrhea, ear infection, pneumonia, and SIDS (Sudden Infant Death Syndrome), among others.

chapter three

So, What Exactly Can My Family Eat?

When a patient first encounters my now-infamous "No, Thank You" list of foods to be avoided on the Plant Paradox program, the most common question I hear is: "What's left for me to eat?"

The honest answer is, a lot of delicious foods! The Plant Paradox plan is not a deprivation diet—it is a roadmap for eating smarter. And while there are certain foods that are off-limits, I've replaced them with healthier versions that will still satisfy your—and your family's—cravings. That means there are substitutes for the carbs you love, like bread, pasta, and pizza; recipe hacks for the tomato-based sauces and condiments you can't live without, like marinara sauce and ketchup; and even decadent, grain- and dairy-free desserts like cheesecake and chocolate chip cookies. Because really, what kid is going to comply with an eating plan that doesn't allow for ketchup and dessert?

And the best part about using a pressure cooker such as the Instant Pot to prepare your meals is that you can still safely eat a number of high-lectin plant-based proteins, such as beans and lentils. I encourage you to embrace the creative food swaps and new preparation techniques in this book, which really do make it easier than ever to eat a low-lectin, high-quality, anti-inflammatory diet. I think you will be amazed at the variety of delicious meals available to you and your family.

Before we get into the details of the "Yes, Please" and "No, Thank You" food lists, I do want to be clear about one thing: There is no way to eliminate every single lectin from your diet, nor would I ever suggest you try to do so—because going entirely lectin-free would mean eradicating all plants from your diet. That's the last thing I want you to do! Some of my critics have mistakenly characterized my program as anti-plant, when nothing could be farther from the truth. You can even be vegetarian or vegan on the Plant Paradox plan. In fact, my wife and I eat a primarily plant-based diet, with a little fish or meat about once a week. My goal is not to scare you away from plants, but instead to arm you with the information you need to choose the best, most nutritious plants possible and to learn some simple cooking methods for reducing their lectin load, so that you can keep your gut buddies happy and your inflammation markers low.

By the way, I've compiled all of these "Yes, Please" "No, Thank You" foods into a handy, at-a-glance list, (pages 57–61). You'll notice the list of "Yes, please" foods is more than twice as long as the list of "No, Thank You" foods—you and your family will not go hungry on this program, I promise you!

Yes, Please: Foods Low in Lectins

FATS

I recommend that between 60 to 80 percent of your total daily calories come from healthy fat sources. That might sound like a lot of fat, and it is—but fat is not something to be afraid of. Contrary to the misinformation about fats popularized by the low-fat diet craze, good quality fats are actually essential for your health, and can even help you lose weight (if that's one of your goals). On the Plant Paradox program, you are likely going to consume more fat than you are accustomed to eating.

What might surprise you is that fats by themselves do not trigger the release of insulin, the hormone that tells your body to store excess sugar and protein as fat. Let that sink in for a moment. Eating fat (without carbs or protein) cannot make you fat. But, the combination of fats with simple carbohydrates (like chips, nachos, fries, or pasta) or fats combined with a lot of protein and carbohydrates (a hot dog or burger with a bun, an order of fries, and a soda) creates the perfect weight-gaining and insulin-pumping storm.

Good fats not only protect and nourish your gut lining,[33] but since your brain is about 60 percent fat, healthy fats improve your and your kids' brain function. The best sources of healthy fats are extra-virgin olive oil, olives, avocados, avocado oil, coconut milk, MCT oil (aka medium-chain triglyceride oil), coconut oil, perilla oil, walnut oil, macadamia oil, algae oil, omega-3 rich egg yolks from pastured hens, and fish oil or algae-based DHA and EPA.

GREENS

Greens contain large amounts of chemicals called polyphenols, which offer many health benefits. Polyphenols act as antioxidants in the body, protecting your tissues against oxidative stress and inflammation and helping to keep diseases like cancer and heart disease at bay. Eating your greens is one of the best choices you can make for your health. In fact, one recent study even found that people who eat a serving of greens a day have a 90 percent reduced risk of developing Alzheimer's disease.[34] Think about it: If we had a drug that effective, how much would you pay for it? Well for about two dollars a day, you can help protect your entire family from cognitive decline. That's one of the best incentives to eat more greens I can think of!

In addition to polyphenols, greens are also rich in fiber, which helps you feel full and keeps blood sugar levels stable. Eating high-fiber foods ensures you are satisfied at meals and aren't hungry between meals, when it's easy to be tempted by less-than-healthy foods.

CRUCIFEROUS AND LOW-LECTIN VEGETABLES

Vegetables should be the focal point of all your meals on the Plant Paradox program, but cruciferous vegetables are particularly beneficial, as they supply nutrition for your gut buddies in the form of prebiotic fiber. Prebiotic fiber cannot be broken down by the digestive enzymes in the gut, and instead serves as fuel for your gut buddies. Prebiotic fiber is literally food for your microbes, and the more you eat, the more they thrive.

Consumption of cruciferous vegetables has also been linked to reduced inflammation. In one study of more than 1,000 women, researchers found that a higher intake of cruciferous vegetables was associated with a 25 percent reduction in inflammation markers.[35] I know inflammation might seem like something that only affects adults, but consider this: Many children today are diagnosed with allergies or asthma, both of which are inflammatory conditions. You have the ability to give your kids the best possible preventive medicine, in the form of the food you prepare for them.

Members of the cruciferous vegetable family include: arugula, bok choy, broccoli, Brussels sprouts, cabbage, cauliflower, collard greens, kale, kohlrabi, Swiss chard, and watercress. Other lectin-free vegetables that offer health benefits are artichokes, asparagus, beets, celery, garlic, leeks, mushrooms, okra, onions, and radishes. One word of caution: if you or your child has IBS, diarrhea, undiagnosed stomach pains or Crohn's disease, or ulcerative colitis, cook these vegetables to "mush" when you first introduce them to avoid digestive distress.

NUTS

Nuts are a terrific source of healthy fats, polyphenols, and fiber. They're great for everyday eating, but portion control is key, as their calorie and protein content can add up quickly. Portable and filling, they make a perfect snack. Keep in mind, not all nuts are compatible with the Plant Paradox program. Peanuts and cashews are legumes and should be avoided. I recommend eating walnuts, pistachios, macadamias, hazelnuts, coconut, chestnuts, blanched or Marcona almonds, and pecans. Be careful with whole almonds if your kids have allergies or autoimmune diseases—the skin on almonds contains lectins that many people react to. Some nuts, like coconut and almond, can also be ground into flour and are great alternatives to wheat flour for baking.

AVOCADOS

Avocadoes are not only delicious, they're also nutritional rock stars. Technically a fruit, avocadoes have no sugar even when ripe and are an excellent source of fat and prebiotic fibers—both of which can help you lose weight and better absorb polyphenols (which are fat soluble) from the plants you eat. Avocadoes are rich in heart-healthy monosaturated fat and, like olive oil, they have been shown to reduce low-density (LDL) cholesterol, aka the "bad" cholesterol.

LECTIN-FREE GRAINS

I realize that it may seem daunting to give up all grains, especially because they are a centerpiece of the American diet and serve as the main ingredient in many people's go-to meals. I'm talking about cereal and oatmeal for breakfast; sandwiches, wraps, and grain bowls at lunch; pasta or rice at dinner—not to mention the many grain-based snacks and sweets we munch on all day. The good news is that today there are so many convenient and tasty substitutes for traditional grains and grain-based flours. In addition, not all grains carry a heavy lectin load: millet, sorghum, and teff are perfectly safe to eat, and even if you haven't tried them before, the recipes in this book will give you everything you need to cook them with confidence. Millet is not only delicious, but is also packed with minerals like magnesium, potassium, and zinc, to name a few. Sorghum, while historically popular in the South, is finally getting the wider attention it deserves. This grain is full of soluble fiber and compounds that are friendly to your gut buddies. Sorghum "popcorn" is a Plant Paradox hack many of my patients love—it smells and tastes exactly like mini-popcorn! Check out the recipe for my delicious and kid-approved Chocolate-Coconut Popped Sorghum on page 204.

RESISTANT STARCHES

Resistant starches are carbohydrates that don't get broken down and converted into glucose as quickly as other types of carbs (like bread for instance—which is almost instantly converted to sugar and then stored as fat in your body). The bulk of resistant starch passes through your intestine intact, because it is more resistant to the enzymes in your gut that break down simple carbs.

This means that eating foods high in resistant starch gives you a (mostly) free pass when it comes to their caloric content and their effect on your blood sugar levels. Your gut buddies also love resistant starches and convert them into important fatty acids that serve as fuel for the cells lining your intestines. In fact, giving your gut buddies the right materials to make more of these fats may be one of the keys to preventing and even healing "leaky gut."

The family of resistant starches includes root vegetables like sweet potatoes and yams, as well as taro root, yucca, green plantains, cassava, tapioca, green bananas, jicama, turnips, and rutabagas, as well as pressure-cooked lentils and beans. Many of these plants have roots that draw water and minerals from the soil for nourishment and possess amazing absorption abilities. High in prebiotic fiber, these are all great sources of fuel for your gut buddies. While it's okay to eat resistant starches daily, if you're trying to lose weight you'll want to be mindful of your portions. If you're cooking for your family, a pound of pressure-cooked lentils will feed everyone under your roof for a couple of meals and will provide excellent nutrition.

WILD-CAUGHT SEAFOOD

Fish and shellfish are some of the tastiest—and healthiest—foods out there. A great source of protein and omega-3 fatty acids, as well as critically important vitamin D, eating wild-caught seafood helps to reduce inflammation, protect you against heart disease, and boost brain health.[36]

But as with most foods, not all seafood is created equal. The seafood I recommend eating must be wild-caught and not farm-raised, even if it is labeled as "organic." Farm-raised fish live in overcrowded conditions, often are treated with antibiotics, and are fed lectin-rich corn and soy, whereas wild-caught fish eat a natural diet of plants, other fish, algae, and so on. And about that "organic" seafood: Do you really believe someone followed the fish around the ocean to see if they ate organically? Of course not! The organic label means they were farmed and fed organic corn, soybeans, or other grains. Though we eat mostly vegetarian or vegan during the week, my wife and I have wild seafood on weekends, both because we enjoy it and because we know it benefits our long-term health. I call this approach to eating "vegaquarian."

PASTURED POULTRY AND OMEGA-3 EGGS

Pastured poultry can be an excellent source of protein and fat. But pastured isn't the same as free-range or organic. In fact, it's critically important to know the difference between these terms when you're selecting proteins for your family. Legally, "free-range" chickens can be kept in warehouses with 100,000 other birds, where they never see the light of day, are fed corn and soy, and are essentially raised no differently than the industrial chicken you've been told to avoid. Pastured poultry, on the other hand, are able to roam and forage for their food—allowing the chickens to fulfill their dietary obligation of eating shrubs, bugs, and grubs. If you're at the grocery store, look for "pastured" or "pasture-raised" on the packaging, or if you're talking to your local farmer at the farmers market, ask him or her how the chickens are raised and fed. (I once asked this question of a farmer at my local farmer's market in Santa Barbara, and she said, "I don't feed my chickens anything, they work for me!" meaning they fed themselves a lot of tasty insects they found on their own.)

Now, a word of warning if you have an autoimmune disease: you may react even to a pastured chicken, as most breeders will supplement some of the chickens' diet with grain-based feed. Just remember that chicken is a modern addition to our diet; your great-grandparents rarely ate chicken; the animals were too valuable as egg layers! Chicken is in no way an essential part of a heathly diet.

As with poultry, I recommend purchasing pastured eggs or omega-3 eggs—the latter designation means that the chickens were fed flaxseeds and/or algae in addition to their normal feed. I actually want you to eat the yolks and limit the whites, as yolks are the part of the egg with the most nutrients and healthy fats. Research has shown that omega-3 eggs can even help lower cholesterol.[37]

ONE HUNDRED PERCENT GRASS-FED MEAT
(AKA GRASS-FED AND FINISHED)

When purchasing meat it's essential to understand what the animal was fed during its life. Sadly, because of poor regulation and misleading labeling, the term "grass-fed" can be applied to animals who were primarily raised on a diet of corn and soy, but fed grass at some point during their lifecycle. Of course, if the animals you're eating ate corn and soy, you're eating corn and soy too. Remember my mantra: You are what you eat, but you are also what the thing you are eating, ate. Most of the corn and soy fed to livestock has been genetically modified, and usually contains even more lectins than their non-GMO counterparts. Moreover, as we discussed earlier, even non-GMO grains and soy are now sprayed with Roundup.

When you're selecting meat, make sure it's not just grass-fed, but also grass-finished. The meat from these animals contains more omega-3 fats and fewer omega-6 fats, the latter of which are easily oxidized and are inflammatory. Good choices include: bison, venison, boar, elk, pork, lamb, beef, prosciutto di Parma, serrano ham, and jamón Iberico. Now let's be clear here: pastured chickens and grass-fed meats are more expensive, often by a lot, compared to the meat farther down the meat counter that may be labeled as "natural" or even "organic." Rather than shrugging your shoulders and saying "I've got to feed my family somehow" while grabbing that cheaper package, I urge you take advantage of the more expensive package as a way to use meat as a side or an accent to your meal rather than putting it at the center of your dinner.

Another thing to consider is that you probably need a lot less animal protein (or any protein for that matter) than you think. We are overproteinized! Yes, it's true that protein is a critically important macronutrient your body needs to build cells and to maintain muscle mass. The amino acids in proteins are literally the building blocks of cells and tissues in the human body—we're made of protein. But in recent years health "experts" and diet gurus alike have overemphasized the importance of protein, and as a result, a lot of people are eating too much of it. Trendy diets like Paleo, Whole30, Keto, Carnivore, and low-carb encourage people to overindulge in protein.

Here's something that is important to understand: the body doesn't waste calories. Any excess protein you eat is immediately converted to sugar, in a process called gluconeogenesis. In most cases, this sugar is then stored as fat. Glucose, as you'll recall from our earlier discussion, also raises blood sugar and insulin levels and lays the foundation for chronic diseases, including type 2 diabetes (which is now at epidemic levels among young people). And adding insult to injury, the amino acids in animal protein appear to be growth agents for cancer and accelerated aging. Beef, pork, and lamb contain sugar molecules called Neu5Gc, which are associated with increased risk of cancer and heart disease. Given these risks, I recommend limiting animal protein intake to no more than four ounces a day.

Though plants contain less protein by weight than animal meat, if you're eating a plant-rich diet, your protein grams will add up pretty fast. An artichoke has about 4 grams of protein, a baked sweet potato, about 2. And so on. Really, if you're eating plenty of plants, you are getting enough protein—so, stop worrying. Keep in mind that some of the largest, most muscle-bound animals on earth eat mostly plants!

Finally, please do not buy into the hype that growing children need significant amounts of animal protein and dairy for proper growth. I assure you, having seen kids all over the world, they grow just fine, and have less incidence of obesity and type 2 diabetes, without prodigious amounts of meats and dairy in their diets.

Calculating Your Protein Needs

So, how much protein should you eat—and do you need more or less than your spouse? What about your kids? How can you make sure everyone in your family is getting enough of those vital building blocks of human life—without overdoing it?

Most protein recommendations are based not on your weight but on your lean body mass, which is difficult to measure. Dr. Valter Longo at the Longevity Institute in Southern California has devised a simpler calculation that I prefer. He and I agree that the average person needs 0.37 grams of protein per kilogram of body weight.[38] To determine how much protein is ideal for you, divide your body weight in pounds by 2.2 to get your weight in kilograms. Then multiply that number by 0.37 and you've got the target number for your daily protein intake.

For kids who are still growing and/or are athletes, you can use the same equation but multiply the final number by 2. So for example, if your 9-year-old soccer star weighs 50 pounds, you would divide by 2.2 to get her weight in kilograms—about 23 kg—and then multiply by .34 to get about 8 grams of protein, and then double it to 16 for her daily intake.

If you're not sure what 16 grams of protein looks like on your plate, in practical matters, it translates to about 2.5 eggs, or a small serving of fish, or a half-cup of tempeh. With animal protein specifically, keep the "one and done" phrase in your head—you don't need to have it at every meal. Try to limit animal protein to a small portion once a day, or spread it out through the day: an egg in the morning, a bit of goat cheese on your salad during lunch, a few shrimp with your dinner. It's easier than you might think for every member of your family to get the protein they need!

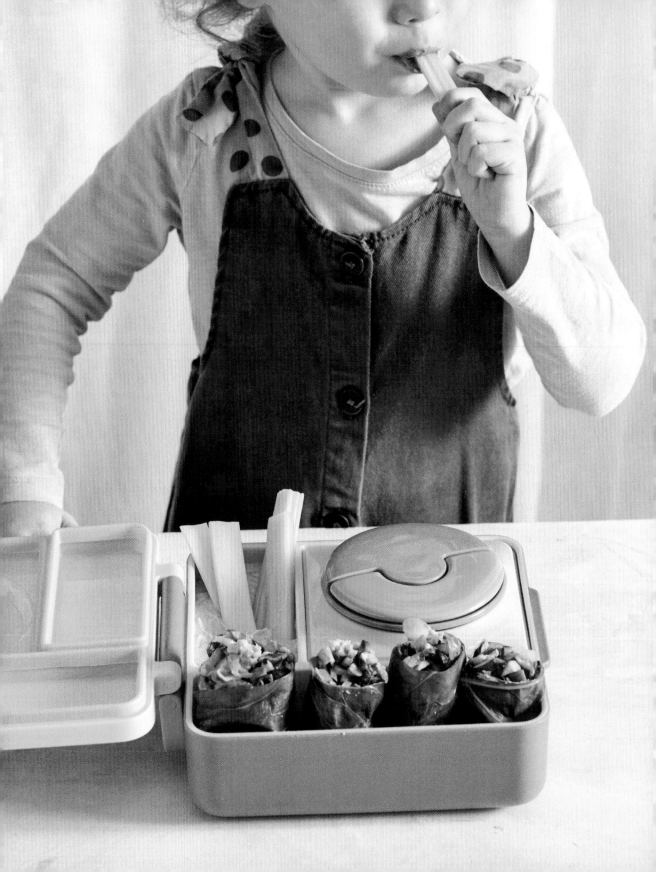

Animal Proteins: What Do All These Labels Mean?

WHEN THE LABEL SAYS...	IT MEANS...
ORGANIC	When it comes to meat, poultry, and eggs, the organic designation means the animals were not fed growth hormones or antibiotics; they were fed organic feed (without GMOs, chemical pesticides, or fertilizers used to grow the grains and soy used in feed); and they were offered the potential for outdoor access (but for only 5 minutes every 24 hours). "Organic" is the only label that requires government inspection and verification. It's a good label to look for when buying meat, but the very best label is "pastured," "grass-fed and finished," or "100% grass-fed." If you observe chickens in their natural habitat, you'll quickly realize that grains and soy are not part of their normal diet, and that cows, whose stomachs are designed to digest grasses, prefer grass to anything else. All of this means that even an "organic" diet is nutritionally lacking and often unnatural for animals.
ALL VEGETARIAN-FED	Found mostly on poultry products, this label means the chickens weren't fed animal byproducts, which likely means that they were given feed that contains grains, pseudo-grains, and/or soy, most of which are loaded with GMOs and lectins. Chickens, which will eat just about anything you give them, naturally prefer insects, so a vegetarian diet isn't actually all that healthy for them!
FREE RANGE	This designation, as codified in a 2007 federal law, means that animals are given access to the outside for at least five minutes a day (yes, you're allowed to scratch your head while pondering this, and yes, five minutes a day is wholly inadequate). "Free-range chickens" typically still live in an overcrowded barn that has some sort of opening—no matter how small—to the outside, although this "outside" can be a small, muddy, fenced-in or netted-in yard, and the barn may be so crowded that most chickens never make it out.
CAGE FREE	While this term may inspire you to envision a bucolic landscape—chickens freely roaming in a grass field—"cage-free" just means that the chickens aren't confined to cages. They are still likely to be confined to an overcrowded warehouse with no guarantee of ever stepping foot outside.

WHEN THE LABEL SAYS...	IT MEANS...
PASTURE -RAISED	"Pasture-raised" hens must be limited to 1,000 birds for every 2.5 acres. That's 108 sq. ft. per bird—approximately 106 sq. ft. more per bird than required for the "free range" designation. Field rotation is mandatory, meaning the hens have to get continual access to grassy fields, not the same area that has already been picked over day and after day by the flock. Also, the hens must be kept outdoors throughout the year—with safe, accessible housing should the hens need to protect themselves from predators, or shelter themselves from extreme weather. When it comes to chicken, pasture-raised really is the highest standard possible.
OMEGA-3	You'll see this term on some egg cartons—it means that the eggs were laid by hens who consume a diet enhanced with flaxseed and/or algae. The polyunsaturated omega-3 fatty acid from the flax and/or algae gets transferred to the yolk when they are digested. In a recent study, omega-3 eggs had approximately 5 times as much omega-3 fatty acid as conventional eggs.[40] Although these chickens likely aren't allowed to forage for their natural diet of grasses, insects, and whatever else they can peck at wandering pastures, omega-3 eggs are often your best alternative if you aren't able to find eggs from pasture-raised chickens, plus they are usually far more affordable than pastured eggs.
HORMONE-FREE	This term, which you'll see on egg cartons as well as labels of poultry and meat, means the animals weren't administered any hormones. However, it doesn't mean they weren't fed lectin-rich or GMO grains, animal by-products, or given antibiotics.
ANTIBIOTIC-FREE	Similar to the "hormone-free" designation, this term means only that the animals weren't given antibiotic injections or had antibiotics added to their feed. It doesn't mean they were fed a natural diet or that they weren't given hormones.
GRASS-FED	Generally used in relation to beef and other animals raised for meat, this designation means the animals were given access to grass at some point in their lives and not that they were exclusively grass-fed. Animals raised for meat are often given hay and access to grass for a little while, then fattened up for slaughter on a diet of grains, antibiotics, and growth hormones. That's why you want to look for meat that either says "grass-fed and grass-finished" or "100% grass-fed."

IN-SEASON FRUIT

Everyone loves fruit, especially kids, and in moderation, it can be a healthy treat and a good source of fiber, vitamins, and polyphenols. But I encourage you to think of fruit more like "candy" than "health food", so please eat it sparingly. And, more important, I encourage you to eat fruit only when in season (remember, naturally ripened fruit contains fewer lectins, whereas out of season fruit, which is picked when underripe, contains more lectins). Our ancestors ate fruit only during the summer months, and the extra calories and sugar allowed them to fatten up for the winter, when food was scarce. Now that fruit is available year-round, we indulge in it 356 days a year, and, unfortunately, signal our bodies to store calories and thus retain fat, all year round. Moreover, fruit today is actually bred for sugar content and size. Blueberries are now the size of grapes, oranges are the size of cantaloupes, and so on.

But, before we get too upset about missing our favorite fruit, the good news is there are some fruits you can enjoy year-round—as long as you eat them before they ripen and are still green (these are the exceptions to the "eat only when ripe" rule!). These fruits include green bananas, plantains, mangoes, and papayas. When these fruits are unripe, they don't contain a great deal of sugar, and our gut buddies feast on their prebiotic fibers. Another way to get the nutritional benefits of fruit without the sugar? Get out your juicer and juice your fruit. Now, throw out the juice and eat the pulp or add it to salads or stir it into baked goods. Or throw it in your blender with some coconut yogurt, a handful of greens, and some almond butter for a gut-friendly smoothie! Here's a time-saving strategy I like to use: Juice your fruit, strain it, and spoon the pulp into silicone ice cube trays and freeze. Pop out the cubes and store in freezer-safe bags. Then, when you are ready, add a few cubes to your smoothie, or even better, stir into coconut yogurt and you will have a healthy fruit "ice cream" in minutes!

CERTAIN TYPES OF DAIRY

As we will discuss in detail in in Chapter 4, most of the dairy products available in the U.S. and Canada use milk from breeds of cows that produce a lectin-like protein known as casein A1, which is converted in your body to the protein beta-casomorphin (BCM). This protein also attaches to the pancreas's insulin-producing cells, known as beta cells, which prompts an immune attack on the pancreas. In addition, most dairy cows are fed a diet of lectin-rich grains and are regularly given antibiotics to treat mastitis infections induced by near-constant milking by heavy machinery. Of course, those lectins and drugs end up in the milk products you consume.

But milk from the cow breeds Guernsey, Swiss Brown, and Belgian Blue do not contain this protein, but rather the protein casein A-2. This type of milk—sold under the label A2 Milk—is becoming increasingly available in stores. In addition to A2 milk, you can safely consume the milk of goats, sheep, and water buffalo. Keep in mind that all milk is an indulgence, as it still contains a lot of sugar. Likewise, you can enjoy, in moderation, cheeses made from goat, sheep, and buffalo, as well as most Italian, French, and Swiss cows.

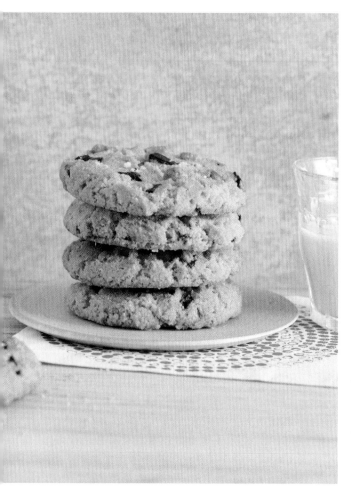

CHOCOLATE

Sometimes, we all get a craving for something sweet, so thank goodness chocolate occupies a space on the "Yes, Please" list!. I think it's important to teach your kids about the true meaning of a "treat," and allowing them to have a small piece of chocolate is a good way to help them understand the ideas of moderation and balance. So long as it's consumed in limited quantities, extra-dark chocolate is a healthy choice. Thanks to cacao—the primary ingredient in chocolate and cocoa—these foods are rich in polyphenols, flavonoids, and fiber, all of which have anti-inflammatory properties Additionally, chocolate is a heart healthy food: as published in the British Medical Journal, eating chocolate may reduce the risk of cardiovascular disease by up to one third![39] When purchasing chocolate, be on the lookout for how much sugar and dairy have been added. Most commercial chocolates are made with tons of added ingredients and do not in any way qualify as "healthy." To get the benefits of chocolate minus the downsides, eat dark chocolate—72 percent cocoa or higher—and limit yourself to one ounce a day or less for you and your kids. That's about one small square (or one of the delicious chocolate chip cookies on page 00!). You can even find chocolate bars sweetened with Stevia and/or monk fruit, sometimes marketed as keto bars, at specialty stores. Be mindful though, when feeding chocolate to children, that it does contains a small amount of caffeine, so, really, all they need is a tiny bit!

No, Thank You: Foods High in Lectins

The Plant Paradox program is based on this one essential axiom: The foods you *don't* eat are far more important to your health than the foods you do eat. Once you remove the inflammatory agents from your diet, your body is able to stop throwing all its resources and energy into dealing with continual damage and instead transition into restoration mode, where excess weight can be shed and diseases can be healed and even prevented.

To that end, what follows is a list of the basic categories of foods excluded from the Plant Paradox protocol. These are foods that no human ate until about 10,000 years ago—and there is no good reason to continue eating them today. Again, you may fast forward to the list on page 59 if you wish, but I think it's helpful to understand why these foods are excluded from the plan. Once you have a sense of the damage these foods can cause, you will be even more motivated to avoid them!

PEANUTS AND CASHEWS

Remember, peanuts and cashews are not nuts: they are legumes loaded with lectins. In fact, the shell that sheaths a cashew is so caustic that workers must wear protective gloves to shell them! In my medical practice, I have witnessed firsthand that eating cashews dramatically increases inflammation, especially in patients with arthritis. Did you know the cashew is part of the same family as poison ivy? I doubt you'd consider munching on that. Since there are plenty of tasty nuts on the "Yes, Please" list, stick to those and your body will thank you. And if you and your kids are die-hard peanut butter fans, I promise you that its tastier cousin, almond butter, is part of the Plant Paradox program.

CORN

Like nearly all other grains, corn (which is not a vegetable, but a grain) has a high lectin content. Corn is one of our country's biggest crops, and it is commonly used as an ingredient in processed foods—think corn syrup, corn starch, corn flakes, corn chips. The average American eats some form of corn multiple times a day.

QUINOA

This New World pseudo-grain is hailed as a healthy gluten-free substitute to wheat, but it is so loaded with lectins that it is no friend to your gut buddies, immune system, or waistline. As for claims that quinoa is good for you because it's an "ancient grain"—yes, it's true that ancient Incas made quinoa a central part of their diet. But what is often missing from this discussion is the fact that the Incas first soaked and then fermented quinoa before cooking it—two instructions you'll rarely ever see on the side of a box of quinoa.

CONVENTIONALLY RAISED MEAT

To understand why corn is among the worst lectin-filled grains, just look at the American farm industry. Farmers use corn for the sole purpose of fattening up cattle. And, guess what? Corn has the same effect on us. Not only that, it causes fatty deposits in muscles. Want well marbled meats? Feed the animals corn. Want your and your kid's muscles well marbled? Cook dinner with conventionally-raised chicken or beef.

Remember, as the chart on page 47 explains in detail, "free-range" meats and chicken won't cut it either. "Free-range" means the cattle and chicken were fed corn, most likely without access to pastures. And therefore, since the protein on your plate ate corn, you are, in essence, eating that corn too. Instead opt for only pasture-raised meats and chicken.

VEGETABLE OILS

You may have heard that vegetable oils are healthier for you than other types of oils, but because most of them are made from high-lectin beans or seeds—such as corn, soybeans, cottonseed, canola seeds, and sunflower seeds—they are all potent sources of lectins. Worse, many of the corn, canola, and soybeans used to make this oil are GMO crops, meaning many of them have been bred to produce extra-strength lectins that help make them more resistant to insects. Additionally, these vegetable oils contain primarily omega-6 fats, so they deliver a double-dose of inflammation when you consume them. I might sound like a broken record, but I'll say it again: all these oils come from grains or seeds sprayed with Roundup, so it too ends up in you!

LEGUMES AND BEANS

Beans, peas, soybeans, lentils and other legumes (also known as pulses) have the highest lectin content of any food group. Is it any wonder that they are also renowned for their tendency to cause gas, bloating, and indigestion?! I know, I know—beans have been hailed as a mainstay of a healthy diet for decades now, particularly if you eat a vegan or vegetarian diet. Don't get me wrong, I am not against legumes and beans! I'm just against eating them without first taming their inflammatory effects. You can dramatically reduce the lectin content of beans and legumes by pressure-cooking them, something we'll cover more in detail soon.

CONVENTIONAL DAIRY

Dairy products made from the milk of most North American cows—even those that are grass-fed and organically raised—contain the lectin-like protein casein A1. The only approved dairy products on this plan are those outlined on page 61, which include A2 milk; dairy products made from goat, sheep, and water buffalo milk; and cheeses from these sources or Southern European cows. The good news here is that coconut milk—the kind that comes in a can as well as the kind that comes in a carton as a milk alternative—makes a great substitute for that creamy dairy taste in soups, ice creams, and other foods.

NIGHTSHADES

This popular family of plants includes potatoes, peppers (bell as well as hot peppers like jalapeño and habañero), eggplant, goji berries, and tomatoes—all of which contain a heaping helping of lectins, in addition to the glycoalkaloid poison, solanine, a known neurotoxin. They are all high in lectins, particularly in their seeds and peels, and therefore unfriendly to your health. Some of my recipes in this book feature tomato sauce; the cooking of tomatoes, and removing their skins and seeds greatly reduces their lectin content.

SQUASH

With the exception of cucumbers, which first originated in Asia and then made their way to Africa and Europe via trade routes, the squash family—fruits with peels and seeds that grow on vines, including pumpkin, acorn squash, zucchini, and butternut squash—are native to the Americas. Meaning, squash contain lectins that humans have only been exposed to in the last five hundred years or so. In addition to containing lectins, squash contain sugars that cue your body to store weight in preparation for winter. All the more reason to not to eat them, or their seeds!

Maybe Foods: Foods with Lectin Count That Can be Reduced with Preparation

Some foods on the "no" list can be made relatively okay in terms of lectins—if you prepare them properly. While I don't advocate eating any of these foods regularly, you can include them in your family's meals occasionally as long as they don't seem to cause you or your children problems (digestive upset, achiness, brain fog, rashes, etc).

BEANS AND LENTILS

For my vegan and vegetarian readers, especially, I know how important beans can be in terms of an affordable fiber-packed, protein-rich food. However, they are loaded with lectins. The good news is that cooking them in a pressure cooker like the Instant Pot all but eradicates their lectin load. Once those pesky lectins are out of the way, beans become the "healthy" food they're often billed as, because your gut buddies love to feast on their soluble fiber.

So if you want to eat beans regularly, I recommend investing in an Instant Pot or other pressure cooker. Yet another bonus of pressure-cooking is that it produces perfectly cooked beans in a fraction of the time it takes to cook them on the stove.

Fermentation is another preparation method that dramatically reduces lectin count. If you want to experiment with this age-old technique, fermenting lentils has been shown to reduce their lectin content by 98 percent.[40] But, word to the wise, this is a technique that takes a good amount of time—and you're probably short on that already, aren't you?

WHEAT AND RICE

The lectin known as wheat germ agglutinin (WGA) is found in wheat bran, which means that whole wheat bread contains WGA, but white bread doesn't. As you may recall, WGA is a nasty lectin—a much smaller protein than other lectins, which means it can sneak through the gut wall even if your gut barrier is fairly healthy. Once freed from your digestive tract and in your bloodstream, WGA wreaks all kinds of havoc—including triggering fat storage, causing neurological problems, and contributing to atherosclerosis.

The positive spin on WGA is that it means delicious, fluffy white bread, naturally raised with yeast or sourdough starters, is better for you than the whole wheat/whole grain stuff marketed as "healthy!" By the same token, brown rice is a whole grain, meaning that white rice (the best choice is basmati rice from India) is actually better for you than brown rice. Let's be clear: while I don't recommend eating wheat or rice, per se, if you're going to eat it, eating the de-hulled versions will reduce your lectin exposure. If you're going to eat white bread, make it even friendlier to your gut by opting for real sourdough, as fermentation also helps reduce the lectin load. And toast it before eating to increase its resistant starch content!

All of that said, if you've been diagnosed with an autoimmune disease or have a family history of them, I recommend avoiding bread in all forms. And please, pressure-cook your white rice! There's no point in trying to pressure-cook wheat in an effort to make it more digestible, as gluten is not destroyed by pressure-cooking. For that reason, there's also no health benefit to pressure-cooking rye, barley, or oats (the other gluten-containing whole grains; even gluten-free oats contain a gluten look-a-like lectin).

TOMATOES, PEPPERS, EGGPLANTS, CUCUMBERS, ZUCCHINI

The first three of these foods are nightshades, which fall under "No, Thank You" on my list. BUT. I know how much people love these foods. Fresh tomatoes are scrumptious and I realize that folks who live in colder climates look forward to tomato season all year long. To make them more digestible, try to stick to heirloom varieties (which have been around longer than most standard varieties and thus, our gut buddies have had at least a smidge more time to acclimate to them) and peel and de-seed them before you eat them. The best way to peel tomatoes is to cut a shallow X on the bottom of them, then drop them in boiling water for a few seconds to loosen the skin. Remove from the water, let them cool, and then the skin will come right off. Then quarter the tomato and scoop the seeds right out. The blanching doesn't affect the taste.

The same goes for peppers of all kinds—peeling and seeding makes them infinitely more digestible. It's easy enough to seed them; to peel them, I like to briefly roast them either on the grill or directly on the burner of my stove until the skin blisters, making it easy to peel off after putting them in a paper bag for a few minutes to steam.

When it comes to cucumbers, zucchini, and eggplant—if you choose to eat these foods, peel them and seed them if possible. "Baby" versions are often easier to work with because they contain fewer seeds. When shopping for eggplant, look for those that have a round bottom as opposed to an oval bottom—they are thought to contain fewer seeds.[41]

THE PLANT PARADOX FOOD LISTS

And now, my friends, I am excited to present to you the part of the book you've been waiting for: The "Yes, Please" and "No, Thank You" lists! Use the lists on the pages that follow as your guide for all food-related questions on the Plant Paradox program. Make photocopies and put them on your fridge. Memorize them as much as possible!

Say "Yes, Please" to These Acceptable Foods

OILS

Olive oil

Algae oil

Coconut oil

Macadamia oil

MCT oil

Avocado oil

Perilla oil

Walnut oil

Red palm oil

Rice bran oil

Sesame oil

Flavored cod-liver oil

SWEETENERS

Stevia (SweetLeaf is my favorite)

Just Like Sugar (made from chicory root [inulin])

Inulin

Yacon

Monk fruit

Luo han guo (aka monk fruit; the Nutresse brand is good)

Erythritol (Swerve is my favorite as it also contains oligosaccharides)

Xylitol

NUTS AND SEEDS
(½ cup per day)

Macadamia nuts

Pili nuts

Baruka nuts

Walnuts

Pistachios

Pecans

Coconut (not coconut water)

Coconut milk (unsweetened dairy substitute)

Coconut milk or cream (unsweetened, full-fat canned)

Hazelnuts

Chestnuts

Brazil nuts (in limited amounts)

Pine nuts

Flaxseeds

Hemp seeds

Hemp protein powder

Psyllium seeds or powder

OLIVES

all

PLANT-BASED "YOGURTS"

Coconut Yogurt (plain)

Pili Nut Yogurt (Lavva Brand)

DARK CHOCOLATE

72% cacao or greater (1 ounce per day)

VINEGARS

all

HERBS AND SEASONINGS

All except chili pepper flakes

Miso

BARS

Adapt Bar: coconut and chocolate (www.adaptyourlife.com)

FLOURS

Coconut

Almond

Hazelnut

Sesame (and seeds)

Chestnut

Cassava

Green banana

Sweet potato

Tiger nut

Grape seed

Arrowroot

ICE CREAM

Coconut milk dairy-free frozen dessert (the So Delicious blue label, which contains only 1 gram of sugar per serving)

"FOODLES"
(my name for acceptable noodles)

Cappello's gluten-free fettuccine and other pastas

Pasta Slim shirataki noodles

Kelp noodles

Miracle Noodle brand pasta

Miracle Noodle Kanten Pasta

Miracle Rice

Korean sweet potato noodles

Palmini Hearts of Palm Linguine

FRUITS (limit all to their seasons except avocado)

Avocados

Blueberries

(continued)

Raspberries

Blackberries

Strawberries

Cherries

Crispy pears
(Anjou, Bosc, Comice)

Pomegranates

Kiwis

Apples

Citrus fruits, lemons and limes
great all year (no juices)

Nectarines

Peaches

Plums

Apricots

Figs

Dates

VEGETABLES

Cruciferous Vegetables

Broccoli

Brussels sprouts

Cauliflower

Bok choy

Napa cabbage

Chinese cabbage

Swiss chard

Arugula

Watercress

Collards

Kohlrabi

Kale

Green and red cabbage

Raw sauerkraut

Kimchi

OTHER VEGETABLES

Treviso, radicchio

Chicory

Curly endive

Nopales, cactus leaves

Celery

Onions

Leeks

Chives

Scallions

Carrots (raw)

Carrot greens

Artichokes

Beets (raw)

Radishes

Daikon radish

Jerusalem artichokes

(sunchokes)

Hearts of palm

Cilantro

Parsley

Okra

Asparagus

Garlic

MUSHROOMS

All

LEAFY GREENS

Romaine

Red-and green-leaf lettuce

Mesclun (baby greens)

Spinach

Endive

Dandelion greens

Butter lettuce

Fennel

Escarole

Mustard greens

Mizuna

Parsley

Basil

Mint

Purslane

Perilla

Algae

Seaweed

Sea vegetables

RESISTANT STARCHES

Tortillas (Siete brand—only those
made with cassava and coconut
flour or almond flour)

Bread and bagels made by Barely
Bread

Julian Bakery Paleo Wraps
(made with coconut flour)

The Real Coconut Café Tortillas
and Chips

Plantain chips
(watch the oils used)

Taro Root chips
(watch the oils used)

Cassava chips and crackers
(watch the oils used)

Jicama chips
(watch the oils used)

IN MODERATION

Green plantains

Green bananas

Baobab fruit

Cassava (tapioca)

Sweet potatoes or yams

Blue or purple sweet potatoes

Rutabaga

Parsnips

Yucca

Celery root (celeriac)

Glucomannan (konjac root)

Persimmon

Jicama

Taro root

Turnips

Tiger nuts

Green mango

Millet

Sorghum and sorghum "popcorn"

Green papaya

Quorn: Meatless Pieces, Meatless, Grounds, Meatless Strips, Meatless Steak-Style Strips, Meatless Turkey-Style Deli Slices only. Don't be confused! These are the only safe Plant Paradox Quorn Products. The rest have lots of lectin-rich ingredients.

Hemp tofu

Hilary's Root Veggie Burger (www.hilaryseatwell.com)

Tempeh (grain free only)

Legumes (or Eden brand canned)

Lentils (preferred)

Black soybeans

Chickpeas

Adzuki beans

Other beans

Peas

The "No, Thank You" List of Lectin-Rich Foods

Pasta

Rice

Potatoes

Potato chips

Milk

Bread

Tortillas

Pastry

Flour

Crackers

Cookies

Cereal

Sugar

Agave

Sweet One of Sunett (acesulfame K)

Splenda (sucralose)

NutraSweet (asparatame)

Sweet 'n Low (saccharin)

Diet drinks

Maltodextrin (okay in tiny amounts)

Peas

Sugar snap peas

Legumes*

Green beans

Chickpeas* (including hummus)

Soy

Tofu

Edamame

Soy protein

Textured vegetable protein* (TVP) (With a proviso here: TVP is pressure extruded under high heat, defatted soy meal; as such it is probably safe lectin-wise, but

use soy with caution due to its estrogen-like effects.)

Pea protein

All beans, including sprouts

All lentils*

Pumpkin

Sunflower

Chia

Peanuts

Cashews

Cucumbers

Zucchini

Pumpkins

Squashes (any kind)

* Allowable for vegans and vegetarians in Phase 2, but only if they are properly prepared in a pressure cooker.

(continued)

Melons (any kind)

Eggplant

Tomatoes

Bell peppers

Chili peppers

Goji berries

NON-SOUTHERN EUROPEAN COW'S MILK PRODUCTS (these contain casein A-1)

Yogurt (including Greek yogurt)

Kefir

Ice cream

Frozen yogurt

Cheese

Ricotta

Cottage Cheese

Butter, unless from A2 cows, sheep, or goats

GRAINS, SPROUTED GRAINS, PSEUDO-GRAINS, AND GRASSES

Wheat (pressure cooking does not remove lectins from any form of wheat)

Einkorn wheat

Farro

Amaranth

Kamut

Oats (cannot pressure cook)

Quinoa

Rye (cannot pressure cook)

Bulgur

White rice

Brown rice

Wild rice

Barley (cannot pressure cook)

Buckwheat

Kasha

Spelt

Corn

Corn products

Cornstarch

Corn syrup

Popcorn

Wheatgrass

Barley grass

OILS

Canola

Corn

Cottonseed

Grapeseed

"Partially hydrogenated" anything

Peanut

Safflower

Soy

Sunflower

"Vegetable"

VEGETABLES

Peas

Sugar snap peas

Legumes

Green beans

Chickpeas (including as hummus)

Soy products

Tofu

Edamame

Soy protein

Textured vegetable protein (TVP)

Pea protein

All beans, including sprouts

All lentils unless pressure cooked

NUTS AND SEEDS

Pumpkin seeds

Sunflower seeds

Chia seeds

Peanuts

Cashews

Acceptable Animal Protein Sources in Limited Amounts

Real Parmesan (Parmigiano-Reggiano)

French or Italian butter

Buffalo butter (available at

Trader Joe's)

Ghee, preferably grass-fed

Goat yogurt (plain)

Goat milk as creamer

Goat cheese, goat butter

Goat or sheep kefir

Sheep cheese and yogurt (plain)

Aged French, Italian, or Swiss cheeses (note, most Swiss cheeses don't come from Switzerland!)

Buffalo mozzarella

Casein A2 milk (as creamer only)

Organic heavy cream

Organic sour cream

Organic cream cheese

Whitefish, including cod, sea bass, redfish, red or pink snapper

Freshwater bass

Freshwater perch, pike

Alaskan halibut

Canned tuna

Alaskan salmon

Hawaiian fish, like mahi-mahi, opakapaka, ono

Trout

Sardines

Anchovies

Smelt

Herring

Mackerel

Shrimp

Crab

Lobster

Scallops

Calamari (squid)

Clams

Oysters

Mussels (farmed okay)

Abalone (farmed okay)

Sea urchin (uni)

Chicken

Turkey

Goose

Duck

Pheasant

Quail

Ostrich

Pastured, non-soy fed, or omega-3 eggs (up to 4 daily), but limit whites, e.g.,

make an omelet with 4 yolks and 1 white)

Bison

Wild game

Venison

Boar

Elk

Pork (humanely raised or pastured)

Lamb (New Zealand is grassfed)

Beef

Prosciutto from Italy

Serrano Ham (Iberico, 5J) from Spain

Bresaola

Liver and other organ meats

Human Food bar

The lists you just read through are quite detailed, and I was joking when I told you to memorize them—there's no pop quiz, I promise! In fact, in the next chapter we are going to break down this list into smaller, more digestible parts...starting with what you need to get in, and out, of your kitchen.

"It Hurts to Walk"

When I met Brian he was a thin, pale 8-year-old boy, whose story was, sadly, all too familiar to me. He'd suffered from multiple ear and throat infections throughout his life (starting as a baby) and had been given many courses of antibiotics to treat them. His hands and feet were covered with red scaly patches that bled when touched. He developed wheezing and was started on asthma inhalers. He complained of "tummy aches" when he ate, and even though he seemed to eat a lot, he was chronically thin. For the last year, his mother had to literally carry him around the house because of his painful, bleeding feet. Multiple specialists suggested his skin condition may be psoriasis and recommended Brian take immunosupressive drugs. His mother sent me some pictures, pleading for help. And help we did!

Blood tests revealed that Brian carried one of the two genes associated with gluten intolerance and had multiple markers for leaky gut and lectin intolerance; his vitamin D level was also horribly low. His parents instituted the Plant Paradox eating program and started Brian on a supplement regimen of pre- and probiotics, vitamin D3, and Omega 3s. Slowly, Brian's weeping, bloody hands and feet began to heal, as I happily discovered through the new pictures arriving in my office every few weeks. Six months later his gut had vastly improved and his bloodwork showed very little evidence of gluten and other lectins in the diet. He could now walk without pain and hold a pen comfotably, and he returned to school. We scheduled his next round of blood tests for 6 months later.

When the time came for me to phone Brian's mother with the results, I was disappointed. Markers of gluten and some leaky gut had returned. Not terrible, but it was there. Expecting the worst, I made the call. To my relief, Brian's mom explained that few days before his blood was drawn, there was a party at school and he was convinced by friends to have a cupcake. Just one. He felt lousy after eating it and didn't want any more. And he hadn't strayed from his diet since! Today Brian is walking on his own two feet again, and breathing easy—his asthma is gone!

chapter four

The Plant Paradox Kitchen

You know that lectins can harm your health, and the health of your family. You know that you've been given incorrect information about your nutritional needs and the nutritional needs of your kids. And you know which foods to eat and which foods to avoid. Now hopefully, you're ready to make some changes.

But where do you start?

Well, everything starts in the kitchen, so before we get to the recipes, let's look go over some quick pantry and kitchen tips to help you get organized. Remember, one of the best strategies for success on the Plant Paradox program is to prepare and plan in advance as much as possible. With that in mind, let's look at how to first purge your pantry of the foods you will no longer be eating, and then how to restock it with high-quality foods and set up your kitchen to make cooking as quick, easy, and pleasurable as possible.

The Pantry Purge

Before you stock your kitchen with delicious, healthy foods, first you have to make space for them by clearing out the junk that's in the way. You probably have a pretty good idea of which foods need to go—bye bye peanut butter; see ya sugary snacks; ciao cereal. While the "No, Thank You" chart on pages 59–60 should be used as a comprehensive guideline, I find it helpful to have a checklist handy as you're sorting through your inventory of food at home. Use it as a reference to help you weed out the main offenders and organize your space, physically as well as mentally. When in doubt, always check labels and look at the ingredients list. Chances are if the list is long, the food is out. If it contains hard-to-pronounce ingredients, it's out. If it contains added sugars, wheat, soy or soybean oil, canola oil, peanuts or peanut oil—it's out.

Items to Toss

Amaranth

Artificial sweeteners

Barley

Bread

Buckwheat

Bulgur

Canola Oil

Cashews

Chia Seeds

Cornstarch

Farro

Flour (all varieties except those listed on page 57)

Fruit, canned

Kasha

Oats/oatmeal

Pasta

Peanut butter

Protein Powder (except those listed on page 57)

Pumpkin seeds

Quinoa

Red pepper flakes

Rice (all except Indian Basmati)

Sunflower seeds

Sugar (all)

Soup, instant or canned

Tomato sauce (jarred)

Vegetable oil

SNACKS

Candy (all!)

Cashews

Crackers (except those listed on page 000)

Cereal

Cookies

Dried fruit (except figs and dates)

Energy bars (except those listed on page 57)

Fruit Snacks

Granola/granola bars

Peanuts

Popcorn

Potato Chips (and all other chips)

Pretzels

Tortilla chips (except those listed on page 58)

Trail Mix

FRIDGE

Beer

Coffee creamer

Dairy products (conventional): milk, cheese, butter, yogurt, cottage cheese

Hummus

Jelly and jams

Juice

Ketchup

Lunch meats

Mayonnaise (unless avocado-based)

Salad Dressing (bottled)

Soda

Soy sauce

Sports/Energy drinks

String cheese

Tofu

Tortillas (except those listed on page 58)

FREEZER

Conventional meat/meat products: chicken, beef, pork, bacon, sausage

Ice cream (unless coconut milk-based with few added sugars)

Microwavable meals

Popsicles and other frozen treats

I know this is a lot to take in. Remember—you don't have to do it all at once. You can edit your pantry and fridge in waves if that's what's most sustainable for your family—just be sure to commit to each wave. Pick a date in advance to tackle a specific area—no backing out! That said, I know that it is not only hard to part with foods you love and rely on—it is also hard part with foods you spent your hard-earned dollars on. I suggest donating unopened items to a local pantry or food bank, so at least you know the food isn't going to waste. For everything else—just do the best you can, as your budget allows. As you remove additional foods over time, you'll make more and more room to add some exciting new ones.

Plant Paradox Pantry Staples

As you make space in your pantry and fridge, the fun part begins: filling it with new foods! Before you get started on your grocery list, I suggest you take a few minutes to read through the summary below of Plant Paradox pantry staples, and then flip through the recipes in Part 2 (page 86) to see which ingredients you might want to stock first. Maybe you can share the book with your kids and let them pick out a recipe or an ingredient they're curious about too. The more they see this lifestyle change as an exciting adventure, the better they will adapt! Here are some of the essential items you'll be using over the next few weeks:

Almond butter: Ideally, you'd purchase organic almond butter made from raw nuts, but if it's too expensive or difficult to find, look for almond butter made without partially hydrogenated oils (aka trans fats) or sweeteners of any kind. You're looking for a maximum of two ingredients: almonds and salt. For those of you with autoimmune disease: look for almond butter made from peeled almonds, like Almondie™.

Almond flour: This flour alternative is made up of only finely ground almonds, which are "blanched," or skinless. It's not the same as almond meal, which usually contains the peels as well. Try to find non-GMO, organic almond flour and store it in the freezer to keep it from going rancid. (Nut flours and nuts, because of their fat content, go rancid at room temperature, so it's best to store them in the freezer or refrigerator.)

Plant Paradox on a Budget

The pantry purge can bring up a lot of mixed feelings, and one very common reaction is some unease about the investment required to shift toward a healthier lifestyle. It is true that some of the foods on the Plant Paradox program are considered specialty items, and organic produce and pastured meats and dairy products are not inexpensive. Over the long haul, you will save money on this plan (on both food and healthcare costs), but in the meantime, as you ease into this lifestyle, here are a few strategies for making your money stretch as far as possible:

- **MAKE A LIST:** And check it twice! Plan your shopping list for each week carefully and stick to it. Scope out sales and deals at grocery stores that stock the foods you need. Recently a number of supermarkets have made a commitment to carry food products and ingredients without artificial colors or flavors, such as Whole Foods and Trader Joe's. Your local stores may have their own organic and in-season sections, but those two are most reliable for me.

- **MEAT ON THE SIDE:** A general rule of thumb in helping to make your dollar go further is to reduce the number of animal products you consume, which is one reason why most of the recipes in this book are or can be adapted to be vegetarian or vegan. If you don't want to completely abstain from meat, I recommend treating it more as a side dish or flavoring rather than the main attraction of your meal. Eating meat in limited quantities will make grocery shopping more affordable.

- **GO WHOLE HOG:** If you do eat meat, one way to get the best quality possible for the lowest price is to purchase a meat share of a pastured animal. Check out your local CSA or farmer's market for information. Typically the smallest purchase is a half or a quarter of an animal, but you can always go in with a few neighbors if you want a smaller amount. To find a local farm that grass feeds and pasture-raises, try a quick internet search, or go to eatwild.com.

- **JOIN THE CLUB:** Join a wholesale club, such as Costco, which is my favorite of the bunch. Aside from my beloved Kirkland Pesto, Costco sells a variety of great items in bulk, including: olive oils, nuts, vinegars, olives, seasonings, dried herbs, spices, Italian butter, organic canned vegetables, broth, and organic frozen vegetables, to name a few. An annual membership in one of these clubs is affordable and will pay for itself over time.

- **SAVE EVERY DROP:** What do you do when you just have a few tablespoons left of a homemade sauce, dip, or condiment that required expensive ingredients (not to mention, time and effort) to make? Scoop the remainder into silicone ice cube trays and freeze, then pop the cubes into freezer-safe bags and label. Those little cubes will come in unbelievably handy when you're preparing meals for younger kids.

- **SHOP ONLINE:** For specialty items that may be harder to find at your local grocery store or wholesale club, sites like Amazon, Thrive Market (which offers qualifying low-income families, veterans, and teachers a free membership), and Vitacost.com are great places to shop.

- **GET YOUR HANDS DIRTY:** Depending on where you live, you can also grow some foods on your own. Herbs are particularly simple to grow and require a minimal investment. Any extra herbs you wind up with at the end of the growing season can be dried and stored. And if you have a little bit more space, consider planting what was once called a "victory garden." Incredibly, during World War II, 40 percent of all the vegetables consumed in America were grown in home victory gardens. Want victory for you and your family is health? It's just outside your back (or front) door!

Almond milk: This milk alternative makes a great substitute in recipes where cow's milk is called for. Look for unsweetened, unflavored versions, and try to find organic and non-GMO brands.

Arrowroot flour: Often labeled as "arrowroot starch," this flour is made from the arrowroot plant's root. It acts as a terrific thickener and works well in sauces where you'd normally use cornstarch. I like to add it to pancake and waffle batters as it helps to hold the batter together.

Avocados: You can't really stock up on enough of these! I recommend eating an avocado a day. To ripen them faster, leave them near your green bananas or place them in a paper bag on your windowsill. If you're really in a pinch, you can put an avocado in a 350°F oven for 10 minutes to soften up. While it won't actually ripen, the texture will at least be softer. Once ripe, avocadoes can be refrigerated for one or two days, or you can peel and pit them, puree the flesh, and then freeze the puree in ice cube trays. I prefer Hass avocadoes, the ones with dark green, lizard-like skin.

Avocado mayonnaise: Mayonnaise is a beautiful, delicious emulsion, but most often store-bought mayonnaise is made with low-quality high-lectin GMO oil, such as soybean safflower, or canola. Mayonnaise made with avocado oil is much better for you. Primal Kitchen makes a great avocado mayo available at Thrive Market and increasingly in regular stores, and you can even find Chosen Foods Avocado Mayo at Costco.

Avocado oil: Boasting a high smoke point and mild flavor, avocado oil is excellent for frying, roasting, and all-around cooking. Costco, Trader Joe's, Whole Foods, and most other supermarkets carry it.

Baking powder (aluminum free): Look for aluminum-free baking powder as aluminum is a neurotoxin. Reliable brands are Bob's Red Mill, Rumford, as well as Trader Joe's and Whole Foods' 365 brands.

Basmati rice: I recommend limiting rice consumption to white basmati rice because it has the lowest lectin content and the highest levels of resistant starch of any rice. Look for basmati rice from India (not Texas, otherwise known as Texmati).

Cassava flour: A popular flour in South American cooking, cassava flour comes from a root known as yucca (or yuca) or manioc, and is full of resistant starch. It is a key ingredient to getting fluffy gluten-free baked goods. If you can't find it in a store near you, look for it on Amazon or Thrive Market (good brands are Moon Rabbit and Otto's Naturals).

Cauliflower "rice:" Riced cauliflower, or cauliflower rice, is just cauliflower chopped up so finely that individual pieces resemble rice granules. You can make it yourself by pulsing the florets in your food processor, or you can purchase it from Whole Foods, Trader Joe's, or Costco. Find it in the freezer section or fresh; it's convenient and cost-effective.

Cayenne pepper: If you love some heat in your food, skip the red chile flakes, which contain skin and seeds of the red pepper (both rich in lectins), and go for cayenne pepper, which is made of ground pepper after it has been peeled, seeded, and dried.

Chocolate: Look for at least 72% cacao when purchasing chocolate; most grocery stores carry some good options, but Costco, Whole Foods, and Trader Joe's are reliable bets. Seek out organic and fair-trade chocolate bars whenever you can, and limit your intake to one ounce (or less) per day; it's a treat, not a necessity. If you're baking, look for an unsweetened, high-cacao content chocolate, with at least 72% cacao. Some products go as high as 99% cacao. Dagoba and Lily's brand also make excellent chocolate chips.

Cocoa powder: This powder is not the same as hot chocolate ("cocoa"), which is a pre-sweetened mix with some cocoa powder and a lot of sugar. Cocoa powder is nothing more than finely ground cacao beans. Because on its own cocoa powder can be fairly bitter (which is actually a good sign, as the flavor is a direct result of all the polyphenols cacao contains), many cocoa powders are "Dutched" and are alkalized with potassium bromate or potassium carbonate to neutralize the taste of the polyphenols. So, if your cocoa powder says "Dutched," skip it, and look for the word "non-alkalized." My favorite cocoa powders are made by Dagoba or Scharffenberger; Trader Joe's also has a non-Dutched variety.

Coconut aminos: Remember how I told you to throw out your soy sauce? Well, this is what you're going to replace it with. Coconut aminos have a similar taste and can be used as a soy sauce substitute in cooking (and for dipping sushi). This product contains only two ingredients: organic coconut tree sap and organic sea salt. You can find it at Trader Joe's, Whole Foods, or online.

Coconut cream: The rich, creamy part of coconut milk, coconut cream lends rich flavor to many dishes. There are two ways to buy it: you can look for cans of coconut cream (I prefer the Trader Joe's brand, but any brand with BPA-free lining will do), or buy coconut milk and refrigerate it overnight. The cream will rise to the top and harden—scoop it out gently the next day, and voila, coconut cream!

Coconut flour: Another great flour alternative, coconut flour helps you make a wide variety of baked goods. Denser than other flours, it absorbs more liquid than you might expect, so make sure you follow recipes to the letter until you get a really clear sense of how this flour works with other ingredients before you do any experimenting on your own. Some of my favorite brands are Bob's Red Mill, Nutiva, and Let's Do.

Coconut milk: Sold either in the refrigerated dairy case in a cardboard carton or the beverage aisle in a Tetra Pak so that it can be stored at room temperature until you're ready to use it, coconut milk is richer than other milk alternatives and works well as a creamy replacement for cow's milk. As you might suspect, I recommend seeking out the unsweetened and unflavored versions.

Coconut oil: Another cooking oil with a high smoke point, coconut oil also makes a great addition to baked goods in place of canola oil or vegetable oil. Look for extra-virgin coconut oil from brands such as Kirkland Viva Labs, Carrington Farms, and Nature's Way.

Eggs: You could say I'm egg-static (sorry, couldn't resist!) about eggs. I advocate the yolks more strongly than the whites, because they are a good source of healthy fats and nutrients. My favorite omelet is made from four yolks and one egg white (you can scramble the excess egg whites and feed them to your pet).

Just make sure you buy eggs that are either pastured or omega-3 enriched, and if buying pastured, look for the soy-free variety.

Erythritol: Your body processes this natural sweetener, a sugar alcohol, differently than traditional sugars, so it doesn't cause a spike in your blood sugar. It's also less likely to cause stomach upset than other sugar alternatives. But the best part: Erythritol acts just like sugar when you bake with it, easily dissolving into batters while retaining great taste. It's often sold under the brand name Swerve; Wholesome sells a version of it too.

Flaxseed meal: Flaxseeds are a great source of short-chain omega-3s and contain no lectins. The only hitch is, they need to be ground in order for your body to be able to absorb those omega-3s, and once ground, they are very prone to oxidation. So the best way to consume flaxseed is to buy whole flaxseeds and grind them as needed in a coffee or spice grinder. If you prefer to buy them already ground, look for a product that was cold-milled, as heat can oxidize the fats, and then store it in the freezer or refrigerator.

Ghee: Otherwise known as clarified butter, ghee is butter that has had the milk solids (which consist of protein, including the troublesome casein A1) cooked and filtered out of it, making it not only shelf stable but also easily digestible. Look for ghee made from the milk of grass-fed cows, which has a higher concentration of omega-3s than conventionally-raised cows. Pure and Pure Indian Foods are two grass-fed brands to look for.

Goat's milk and goat's milk cheese and yogurt: Goat's milk doesn't contain casein A1 and so is a gut-friendly alternative to conventional cow's milk. More important, if you are using animal milk to feed your baby or children, goat's milk is more similar to human milk than cow's milk. (It's no wonder goat's milk has traditionally been called "mother's milk") You can also use goat cheese, sometimes labeled as "chèvre," and goat's milk yogurt or kefir (purchase unsweetened, unflavored varieties) in your cooking. Thankfully we are now also seeing goat's milk used as a base for cheeses like cheddar and mozzarella, making it easier to cook your and your kids' favorite foods.

Hemp milk: The same hemp that is kin to marijuana (although eating or drinking it will not give you a high), hemp milk is yet another alternative to cow's milk that's great in smoothies and other recipes. I know I sound like a broken record, but stick to the unsweetened, unflavored varieties.

Hemp protein powder: A great alternative to whey or pea protein powder for vegans or anyone else who wants to reduce their intake of animal protein, hemp protein powder provides all the essential amino acids and plenty of omega-3s. Trader Joe's reliably carries it in their stores.

Hemp tofu: Another way to enjoy the nutritional benefits of hemp is with this more densely textured alternative to traditional tofu, which is made from soy beans and is high in lectins. You can find the non-GMO brand Living Harvest Tempt hemp tofu at Whole Foods.

Honey: Although honey is a "natural" sugar, it is still sugar and should be consumed only in very small amounts—one teaspoon or less a day. Honey contains enzymes that provide health benefit that no other natural sugar can match, but sugar is sugar. If you need a sweetener and for some reason stevia, erythritol (Swerve), or monk fruit just won't cut it, you can use a little bit of raw local honey (which contains beneficial organisms) or Manuka honey (which has antiviral and anti-inflammatory benefits). For the record, pasteurized honey is essentially sugar syrup and unless you cannot consume raw honey, you should not purchase the pasteurized variety.

Inulin: Sold under the brand name Just Like Sugar, inulin is made from chicory root or agave (the plant used to make tequila) and is useful in baking and in regular cooking as a replacement for sugar. It provides your gut buddies with a fructo oligosaccharide you can't digest, but they love. You can also find it at Whole Foods under the brand name Viv Agave Organic Blue Agave Inulin, or online.

Millet: You're probably familiar with millet as it is a popular component of birdseed. But it's not just for the birds! This hull-less (and thus, lectin-free) grain is a tasty addition to your diet and can be used as a stand-in for rice or quinoa in grain bowls.

Miracle Rice: If you're really missing your rice and eating a small amount of white Basmati rice just isn't going to cut it (and you don't want to burn out on cauliflower rice), try this "rice" made from the lectin-free konjac root. You can find Miracle Rice in the refrigerated section of most grocery stores, near the tofu.

Mozzarella: True buffalo mozzarella—the kind that comes in ball-shapes of different sizes—is made from the milk of water buffalo, meaning it doesn't contain casein A1. Read labels carefully; "buffalo milk" should be the main ingredient. Most shredded mozzarella that comes in re-sealable bags is made with cow's milk. (You can also find goat's milk mozzarella at Whole Foods or on Amazon.)

Nori: If you're missing the convenience of tortillas, try this seaweed product that is often used in sushi rolls and is about the thickness of a sheet of paper. It makes a great wrap for scrambled eggs, tuna or salmon salad, or other sandwich fixings. Look for organic nori.

Nutritional yeast: This is not the kind of yeast that causes bread to rise; it's a B-vitamin-rich powder that lends a savory, cheesy taste to anything you sprinkle it on. I use it on my Cheesy Almond Crackers (page 172). Nutritional yeast is available in natural food stores, grocery stores like Whole Foods, or online.

Olive oil: I prefer Mediterranean olive oils, especially Moroccan, Italian, Greek, and Spanish olive oils, but there are also some great American olive oils like "O," Bariani, and California Olive Ranch. Make sure to buy extra-virgin—I get mine at Costco, the Kirkland label, which comes from Tuscany. If you can find (and afford) organic, that's your best choice. Good olive oil should be noticeably green, have a fresh, grassy smell, and come in an opaque glass bottle because light causes it to deteriorate. By the way, if the oil makes you cough when you first try it, that's a good thing—it's a sign that it's rich in polyphenols! Always look for a pressing date—the oil goes bad about a year after that.

Paprika: This is another pepper-derived spice, like cayenne pepper, that doesn't include the skins and seeds and is therefore low-lectin. Smoked paprika in particular imparts a rich flavor to a variety of dishes and is especially delicious in stews and chilis.

Parmigiano-Reggiano: The real deal Parmesan cheese, made from the milk of Italian cows—which doesn't contain casein A1 is produced only during the spring and fall, when grasses are abundant (the cows are grass-fed). It can cost up to $20 per pound, but just a little bit of this strong, salty cheese packs a big punch. Hold onto the rinds once the cheese is mostly used and add them to your broths, stocks, and soups to add depth of flavor.

Pecorino Romano: This Tuscan grating cheese is made from sheep's milk and has rich, nutty flavor that pairs well with pasta dishes. Like with Parmesan cheese, just a few pinches adds a lot of flavor to a dish.

Perilla oil: This oil, made from the seeds of the perilla plant, is the most common cooking oil used in Asian countries. It is a great source of the omega-3 fat alpha linolenic acid—containing more of it than any other oil. It also contains rosmarinic acid, which benefits brain health. I didn't call for perilla oil in the recipes in this book, but it can be used interchangeably with olive oil or coconut oil. Look for it in Asian markets, natural food stores, and Whole Foods.

Quorn products: This is a meat substitute derived from mushrooms, but it doesn't taste as "meaty" as mushroom; it's more similar in taste and texture to chicken. Not all Quorn products are Plant Paradox–friendly—stick to the tenders, cutlets, and ground versions. It's important to note that these products aren't vegan—there's a little egg white protein in them. The products in the vegan line contain potato and gluten, so they aren't part of the Plant Paradox program. Stay away from any breaded varieties as well. You can find Quorn products in the vegetarian freezer section of most supermarkets.

Sea salt, iodized: Sea salt contains many more trace minerals than traditional table salt and is therefore much more healthful. However, be sure to look for versions of sea salt that contain added iodine. Iodine is essential to thyroid function, and the most typical way we get it is by eating iodized table salt. Once the foodie craze kicked in and so many people switched from traditional table salt to sea salt, doctors like myself started to see iodine deficiencies become more common. So give yourself the best of both worlds and buy iodized sea salt. It's pretty easy to find in most supermarkets, and even Morton's now produces an iodized sea salt.

Sorghum: Along with millet, sorghum is one of the few grains without a hull. It can be eaten as a breakfast cereal, served as a side dish, or even popped like popcorn. Bob's Red Mill carries it, or you can find a popped version of it, called Mini Pops, online.

Stevia: This natural sweetener contains no calories and won't cause a spike in blood sugar. Derived from the stevia plant, you can buy it in powdered form or in liquid drops. Because it is 300 times sweeter than sugar, a little bit goes quite a long way. I prefer the SweetLeaf brand because it doesn't have fillers such as maltodextrin like other brands often do, and the first ingredient is inulin, which your gut buddies love.

Tempeh: Tempeh is a form of fermented soy. You can find it at the supermarket in the refrigerator case by the tofu. Look for organic, non-GMO versions (as most soy is GMO) made without grains. Please be careful though, most tempeh sold in the U.S. is mixed with grains. Like tofu, tempeh doesn't have a great taste on its own, but picks up the flavors of other ingredients well, and is a good source of protein for vegans and vegetarians.

Vanilla extract: Be careful to only buy vanilla extract that says "pure" on the label—otherwise, what you're buying likely contains a slew of chemicals that mimic the taste of vanilla rather than the beans themselves. If you are missing sweetened, flavored yogurts, add a touch of pure vanilla extract and a few drops of stevia to your goat, sheep, hemp, or coconut yogurt—kids love it too.

Walnuts: Walnuts are rich in fiber, protein, and essential fatty acids. In fact, research has shown that consumption of just two ounces of walnuts a day for about two weeks, significantly affected the growth of tumors in confirmed breast cancers, and thus raised chances of survival.[46] Look for organic walnuts, and for a longer shelf life, keep them refrigerated.

Yogurt: Look for yogurt made from goat's, sheep's, hemp, or coconut milk. You can find a wide variety of these yogurts at Whole Foods, Trader Joe's, and natural food grocery stores. Just be sure to read labels carefully and be on the lookout for added sugars—choose "plain" options.

Plant Paradox Kitchen Tools

In addition to clearing out and restocking your pantry, I recommend taking a little time to clean out, organize and, if necessary, supplement your kitchen tools. While I usually don't suggest that any specialized cooking equipment is necessary to follow the Plant Paradox program, given the focus of this book, I do recommend you invest in either an Instant Pot or a slow cooker to help make your life easier and get dinner on the table faster. Below is a full list of the kitchen equipment that will make food preparation simpler, and your time in the kitchen more enjoyable. As with the pantry overhaul, there's no need to rush out and buy everything at once—go slowly, and only purchase new items as needed. Keep an eye out for sales and specials around holidays (Black Friday sales are some of the best for cookware, and in May cookware is often discounted again), and do your research online to find the best prices.

Blender: I use my blender nearly every day. High-speed blenders such as Blendtec, Vitamix, or Ninja make quick work of smoothies, can blend and heat soups (so no need to dirty a pan), and do some of your prep work for you by chopping and combining ingredients. If you don't have a full-size blender and don't want to acquire one, the Magic Bullet or the larger NutriBullet are good, smaller options.

Food Processor: A food processor is like having three extra sets of hands. It chops, mixes, and slices in just a few pulses. And you'll never again have to scrape down the sides of a blender when making pesto or other sauces!

Ice Pop Molds: If you have young kids (and even if you don't!), healthy ice pops are easy-to-make treats that stay fresh in the fridge for a week or more. I recommend using silicone molds, which release the pops easily and are dishwasher-safe, but make sure that any molds you use are BPA-free.

Instant Pot or other pressure cooker: If you want to enjoy eating beans, lentils, or tomato sauce—as well as cut down on cooking time and cook in larger batches for a family—a pressure cooker is an essential cooking appliance. I love the Instant Pot, which regulates the pressure for you, so you don't have to worry about a thing. You can also use the Instant Pot as a slow cooker, or as a sauté pan (it has a high-heat setting so you can brown meat or onions right in it). Just be sure not to overfill any type of pressure cooker, digital or not. That "do not fill above this line" line is not a suggestion, it's a rule for your safety.

Knives: A good chef's knife and paring knife makes vegetable prep a breeze. Keep them well-sharpened as you are more likely to injure yourself with a dull knife than a sharp one. Good knives are a cook's best friend.

Magic Bullet: This mini appliance is a blender/food processor hybrid. It's great for single-serving foods like smoothies, but if you are cooking for a family, you would probably be better served with a full-size high-speed blender.

Microwave: You probably already have one of these, but if you don't, there's certainly no need to purchase one. That said, they do come in awfully handy for thawing frozen leftovers and reheating last night's dinner for lunch the next day.

Mixing Bowls: The right mixing bowls can make a huge difference in your ease and enjoyment of cooking. Look for a set (large, medium, and small) with high sides so ingredients don't slosh over the edge and onto your countertop or floor when you're mixing. I recommend using glass bowls, but if buying another type of bowl, please avoid plastic.

Salad Spinner: I know what you might be thinking—not another bulky gadget! But greens are central to the Plant Paradox plan, and if they are cleaned and dried properly they will last longer in the fridge and cut down on prep time when you're cooking. I could not believe the difference this gadget made in my, and my wife, Penny's, lives! It makes it so much easier to have organic greens and lettuces at the ready anytime: just chop, throw in the spinner basket, rinse, then spin away the water! No more plastic bags that use questionable chemicals to keep that pre-chopped lettuce "fresh" for days!

Sheet pan: A number of recipes in this book utilize a sheet pan to create easy, "one and done" sheet-pan suppers. You probably already have a few of these—and they are likely old and covered with years of charred residue. I suggest purchasing a new rimmed sheet pan with a ceramic coating—you can find them online for about $20. And for ease of cleanup (and keeping your pan looking like new), line the pan with parchment paper when cooking any foods that don't need to be crispy (the parchment will absorb moisture).

Skillets: A good-quality pan that evenly distributes heat makes food taste better and makes cleanup easier. Please resist the temptation to buy or use a skillet with a nonstick coating, as these contain dangerous chemicals that leach into your food. Instead, look for a skillet with a ceramic coating or made from high-quality stainless steel. And please, throw away that cast iron skillet without a ceramic coating. I can't tell you the number of patients I see who use a cast iron skillet about once a week and have dangerously high iron levels.

Slow Cooker: A number of recipes in this book can be prepared using a slow cooker, which is another appliance that minimizes your time in the kitchen. Slow Cookers are a worthwhile investment for busy families and working parents with long hours. Just throw a few ingredients into the slow cooker in the morning, turn it on, and dinner is ready when you get home.

Spiralizer: This handy tool makes noodles out of all kinds of vegetables, such as jicama, sweet potatoes, and daikon radish, so you can enjoy "pasta" minus the lectins. You don't need a fancy, electronic one. The hand-held version works just fine and costs about $15.

Vegetable Peelers: Remember, lectins are found in the peels and seeds of plants, so having a peeler helps you lighten your lectin load. I recommend having two kinds: One with straight-edge blades and one with serrated-edge blades. The serrated edge lets you peel delicate foods, like tomatoes, saving you the step of blanching them.

Meal Planning 101

Now that your kitchen is cleaned out and ready to go, it's time to start on your grocery list. But before you can write a list you need to know your game plan—or meal plan—for the week ahead. If you're not someone who typically plans out each meal of the week, don't panic: You're not alone. A lot of busy families are playing it by ear, cooking meals on the fly, or not planning out more than a day ahead. But not only will planning a week (or more) of meals make it easier to stay on the program, it will also save you time and money.

The best way to get going on your meal plans is to flip through the pages in the recipe section of this book and select those that most appeal to you. Then compare the ingredients lists—are there recipes that utilize the same ingredients, thus minimizing the items on your shopping list? Which ones would make the best leftovers for lunch? (Hint: braised foods like stews and chilis are perfect for packing into a thermos the next day.) Which recipes do you think you might want make a double batch of and freeze for future meals?

To get you started, I've put together a few sample plans that take these questions into consideration. Feel free to mix and match based on your family's needs and preferences, or follow the plan as is to get started. I didn't account for snacks and treats here, because I don't recommend eating in between meals and indulging in treats on a daily basis. But you can plan for your snacks in the same way you would meals—hard-boiling half a dozen eggs for on-the-go snacking, or baking a dozen cookies or making a batch of ice pops for treats that will last a week or more.

Finally, a note about meal planning for those who are looking to lose weight or see dramatic results. I do recommend intermittent fasting as part of the Plant Paradox program, for adults only, but given the focus of this book, I've chosen not to include a fasting protocol here. If you'd like to learn more about the benefits and practice of intermittent fasting, you can turn to *The Plant Paradox* or *The Plant Paradox Quick and Easy* as a resource. In the meantime, just know that prolonging the time your digestive system has to rest between meals offers many health benefits—so when you'd like to, feel free to skip breakfast and eat an earlier dinner. You can customize your meal plan to suit your and your family's needs!

Sample Meal Plans

DAY	BREAKFAST	LUNCH	DINNER
DAY 1	Breakfast Casserole for a Crowd (page 92); save leftovers	Lettuce Wrap "Tacos" (page 178)	Sheet Pan Turkey Dinner (page 118)
DAY 2	Green Banana Bread (page 93); save leftovers	Thanksgiving Sandwich (page 163) made with leftover turkey	Portobello "Pot Roast" (page 140) with "Baked" Sweet Potatoes (page 237)
DAY 3	Breakfast Casserole for a Crowd (leftovers)	Portobello "Pot Roast" (leftovers)	"Spaghetti" and Meatballs (page 134); save extra sauce
DAY 4	Shakshuka (page 97) with tomato sauce (leftovers)	Vegetable Roll-Ups (page 168)	Green Chili with Chicken (page 153)
DAY 5	Green Banana Bread (leftovers) or hardboiled egg with avocado slices	Green Chili with Chicken (leftovers)	Cauliflower Broccoli Nuggets (page 112) with Five-Minute Brussels Sprouts Salad (page 183)
DAY 6	Sweet Potato Egg Nests (page 101)	Five-Minute Brussels Sprouts Salad (leftovers), Lectin-Free Lunch Kits (page 171)	Not-Too-Spicy Tikka Masala (page 132) with Keto Naan Bread (page 184)
DAY 7	Coconut Mochi Pancake (page 90); save leftovers	Not-Too-Spicy Tikka Masala (leftovers) with cauliflower rice	Clean out the fridge night— everyone picks their favorite leftovers from the week!

DAY	BREAKFAST	LUNCH	DINNER
DAY 8	Hot Breakfast Cereal (page 89)	Lectin-Free Lunch Kit (page 171) and green salad	Cauliflower "Mac" and Cheese (page 115) and green salad
DAY 9	Coconut Mochi Pancake (leftovers)	Egg, Tuna, or Hearts of Palm Salad (page 166–167) sandwich with Sturdy Sandwich Bread (page 164); save leftover bread for the week or cut into slices and freeze	Bean and Mushroom Chili (page 154) with "Baked" Sweet Potatoes (page 237)
DAY 10	Toast made from Sturdy Sandwich Bread (leftovers) with Seasonal Fruit Jam, grass-fed butter, or almond butter	Bean and Mushroom Chili with "Baked" Sweet Potatoes (leftovers)	Sheet Pan Fajitas (page 122) with guacamole and steamed cauliflower rice
DAY 11	Hot Breakfast Cereal (page 89); save leftovers	Sheet Pan Fajitas (leftovers)	Hearts of Palm "Fish" Sticks (page 129), Instant Pot Okra (page 195), green salad
DAY 12	Avocado toast: Sturdy Sandwich Bread (leftovers), toasted, with avocado, a squeeze of lemon, and a sprinkle of sea salt	Hearts of Palm "Fish" Sticks, Instant Pot Okra, green salad (leftovers)	Perfect Roast Chicken and Vegetables (page 142)
DAY 13	Hot Breakfast Cereal (leftovers)	Perfect Roast Chicken (leftovers) over greens with avocado	Thai Coconut Chicken (page 146) with Perfect Basmati Rice (page 231)
DAY 14	Shakshuka (page 97), with Sturdy Sandwich Bread (if there is any leftover) on the side for dipping	Leftover Thai Coconut Chicken or Vegetable Roll-Ups (page 168)	Clean out the fridge night—everyone picks their favorite leftovers from the week!

The 4 Rules

Now that you're ready to dive into the kitchen and get cooking, let's take a moment to review the basics of the Plant Paradox protocol. The entire philosophy of this program can be summarized in the following four rules:

RULE 1: What you remove from your diet has a far bigger impact on your health than what you add to it.

This isn't a nutrition plan focused on the latest "miracle" foods. After twenty years of clinical research with my patients, many with children and teenagers with severe asthma, eczema, allergies, and autoimmune diseases, I am telling you that what you remove from your and your kids' diets will have a far more positive impact on your and their health than what you add to it. If all you did was ditch the foods on the "No, Thank You" list on pages 59–61, you and your family would notice improvements immediately. There's a reason I list this rule first; and it's because it's the most important one!

RULE 2: Take care of your gut buddies and they'll take care of you.

You've likely been waging a full-on battle with the microbes in your gut for a long time. Between taking medications like ibuprofen and other non-steroidal anti-inflammatory drugs, antibiotics, and antacids, as well as eating a diet that includes pesticide-treated foods, processed foods, and foods that are high in sugar and saturated fats, your gut buddies have been struggling to hang in there. But when you stop consuming these substances, the microbes that are so vital to your wellbeing will begin multiplying in droves. Here's how I like to look at it: When you start eating the foods that nourish your gut buddies and allow them to proliferate, you become healthier, mentally sharper—like a superhero version of yourself! As Bette Midler would say, your gut buddies become "the wind beneath [your] wings."

RULE 3: Fruit = Candy.

I know this is a tough one, so it bears repeating: please think of fruit as a treat to be enjoyed in moderation, not as a health food to be consumed regularly. Yes, fruit contains nutrients, polyphenols, vitamins, and fiber—but so do vegetables, minus the sugar. The sugar content in fruit is particularly troublesome. The sugar in fruit is fructose, which is especially appealing to cancer cells—it's their preferred source of fuel.[42] All sugar (fruit and non-fruit) causes a spike in blood sugar and insulin, which triggers an inflammatory response from your immune system. I liken eating a bowl of fruit for breakfast to eating a bowl of Skittles—and would you ever let your kids eat candy for breakfast? Of course not. It also bears repeating that juice—fresh squeezed or otherwise—is just concentrated sugar water.

In addition, much of the fruit we eat is shipped across long distances and thus must be firm to hold up in transit—so it is harvested before fully ripening. This means that the peels and seeds have a high lectin concentration. So when you do eat fruit, it's important to choose locally grown, in-season fruit to minimize lectin exposure. Also remember that a "fruit" is classified as any produce item that contains seeds (the exception to this rule is strawberries, the sole fruit with seeds on the outside).

It is true that some nutrients, like polyphenols, are found only in specific fruits (like resveratrol in the skin of red grapes). But green and cruciferous vegetables contain many other important polyphenols and nutrients and are much more beneficial for your overall health. Bottom line: When you reduce fruit consumption, your family's nutritional needs will be met just fine, as long as everyone eats their vegetables!

RULE 4: You are what the thing you are eating, ate.

If you and your family choose to eat animal protein, it's important to keep in mind that eating any meat other than wild-caught seafood and pasture-raised chickens, cows, lamb, and pigs (or any other animal you eat) means that you are also eating some nasty chemicals, as well as lectins. Conventionally- and even organically-raised animals are fed a diet of corn, soy, and/or wheat, ingesting a ton of lectins, which in turn, are ingested by you and your family. If you remove all other high-lectin foods from your diet but still eat conventionally-raised animals, you are, in fact, sabotaging yourself. Yes, pastured meat is costly, so just do the best you can. My preference is to treat meat as more of a weekly indulgence than an everyday necessity, so I feel comfortable splurging on the best quality I can find.

Okay, enough with the preparation already: It's time to eat! In Part 2, you'll find recipes for every meal of the day, as well as vegetable-focused side dishes, lunchbox-friendly meals for little kids (and big kids!), and even some indulgent desserts. Many of these meals can be made with an Instant Pot or slow cooker, while others are simple sheet pan meals that require very little prep and hardly any dishwashing. If you don't have an Instant Pot or slow cooker, don't worry. You can adapt these recipes to make them on the stovetop as well—they will just require a little bit more cooking time.

Are you ready to get cooking? Let's go!

A Baseball Cap to Hide Her Pain

Regina was a beautiful, smart, totally bald 6-year-old girl whose parents brought her to see me after the treatments she'd received for alopecia areata had failed to help her. The family had been told that all trials of steroids and immune-suppressing drugs hadn't worked. When I met her, she wore a baseball cap that had a fake blond ponytail coming out the back. Even her eyelashes were gone.

Blood work revealed she had an anti-histone antibody that was a marker for an autoimmune disease similar to Lupus. I instructed her and her parents on the Plant Paradox protocol, and started her on vitamin D and omega-3 supplements. We met again three months later. Her Histone marker was down, her Vitamin D and Omega 3 levels were coming up, and she had about an inch of "peach fuzz" on her scalp and the beginnings of eyebrows. We were all delighted! After another three months of following the plan, her Histone returned to normal and she had several inches of healthy hair growth on her scalp! The baseball cap was gone.

We elected to see her six months later, but before that appointment, I received a frantic email from Regina's mother with a new picture: her hair had completely fallen out again. Repeat blood tests showed her Histone was again positive; the family came back into see me early, and this time the baseball cap was back on. On questioning, Regina told me and her parents that when at school or visiting friends' houses, she had been convinced to "cheat" with the occasional cookie or glass of milk or even a sandwich. After all she was a normal 7-year-old kid.

But despite the temptations, Regina was determined to commit to the plan and regrow her hair. Her parents talked with the school, which allowed her to bring her own food from home. They also spoke with the parents of Regina's friends so that everyone could be aware of the rules moving forward and help to support Regina. I'm happy to report that, as of this writing, Regina's hair is once again growing in. I hope she can get rid of that baseball cap once and for all.

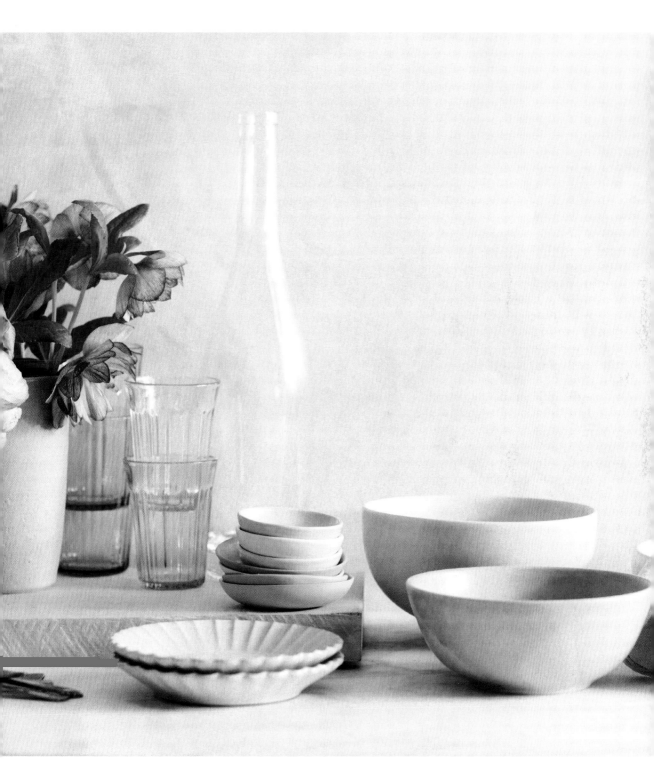

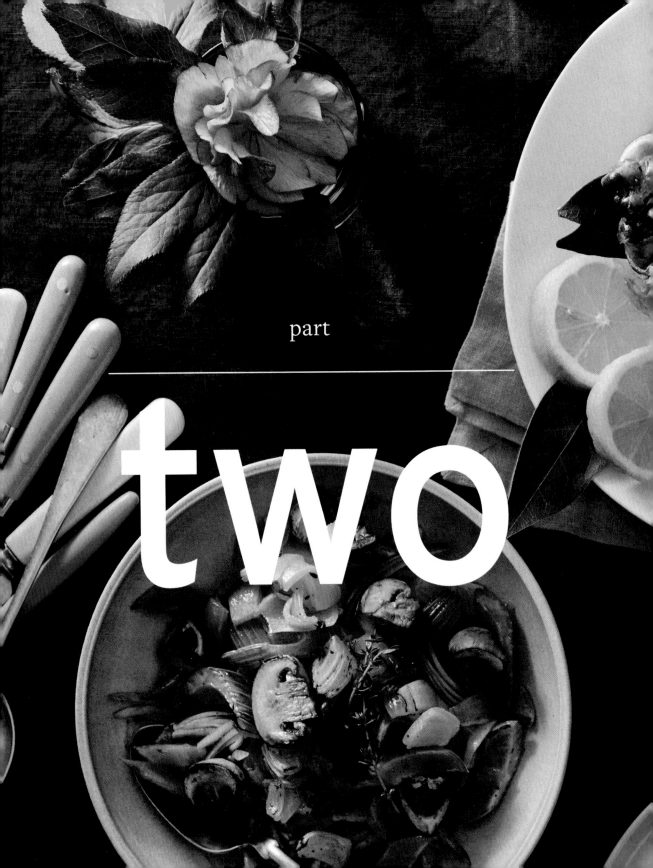

part

two

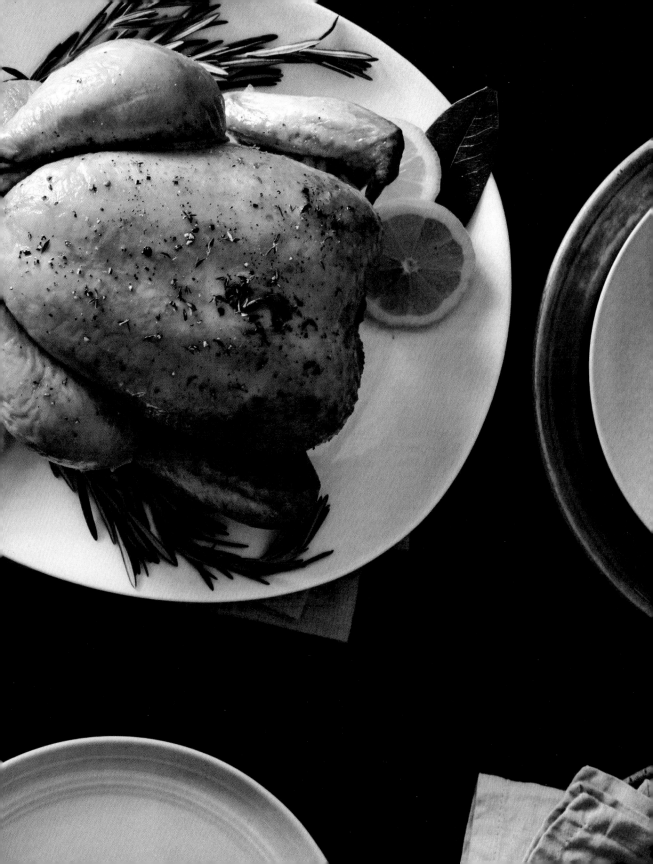

chapter five

Breakfast Made Simple

Hot Breakfast Cereal

While oats are not Plant Paradox–compliant, millet makes an excellent stand-in for a simple and satisfying hot cereal. Made with figs, nuts, and a fragrant blend of warming spices, this is a nutritious breakfast every member of the family will enjoy. Pressed for time? Prepare it the night before, portion out into mason jars, and reheat in the morning with a splash of coconut milk or water!

SERVES 4 TO 6

1½ cups uncooked millet

2 cups water

1 cup coconut milk

½ cup unsweetened shredded coconut

¼ cup monk fruit sweetener (optional)

1 teaspoon cinnamon

½ teaspoon nutmeg

¼ teaspoon cloves

¼ teaspoon allspice

½ teaspoon sea salt

½ cup minced dried figs (optional)

½ cup minced toasted walnuts

1. Set your Instant Pot to sauté, and toast the millet, stirring frequently, until it smells nutty.

2. Add the water, coconut milk, shredded coconut, sweetener, if using, the cinnamon, nutmeg, cloves, allspice, and salt, and cook on high pressure for 10 minutes.

3. Allow the pressure to release manually. Uncover, and add the figs, if using, then put the cover back on. Let the figs sit and hydrate in the cereal for 10 minutes.

4. Fold in the toasted walnuts, and serve.

Coconut Mochi Pancake

This light, sticky cake rises from a lush batter of coconut yogurt and almond milk steamed in an Instant Pot. The texture is different than a traditional pancake—think spongey rather than fluffy—but I find it addictive. Try serving with a portion of in-season fruit or some coconut cream for a breakfast that feels like a special treat.

SERVES 4 TO 6

100% olive oil or avocado oil cooking spray (used twice)

4 large omega-3 eggs

Juice and zest of 1 large lemon

1 tablespoon vanilla extract

2 tablespoons avocado oil

⅔ cup monk fruit sweetener

1½ cups unsweetened coconut yogurt

½ cup coconut milk or unsweetened almond milk

½ cup millet flour

½ cup tapioca flour

½ cup blanched almond flour

½ teaspoon sea salt

1 teaspoon baking powder

½ teaspoon baking soda

½ teaspoon allspice

Fresh fruit or sliced figs (optional)

1. Spray a cake pan that fits into your Instant Pot with oil. Both 6- and 7-inch springform pans work well; a 6-inch pan produces a thicker cake, like the one in the photo here. Place the trivet in the Instant Pot and add 1½ cups water to the pot.

2. In a high-speed blender, add the eggs, lemon juice and zest, extract, avocado oil, sweetener, yogurt, and milk, and blend until smooth.

3. In a small bowl, whisk together the millet, tapioca and almond flours, salt, baking powder, baking soda, and allspice until very well combined and clump free.

4. Add the flour mixture to the blender and blitz until smooth. Set aside, and let the flours hydrate for 5 minutes.

5. Spray your Instant Pot thoroughly with oil or line with parchment paper, then pour the batter into the prepared pan, and place in the pot. The batter should fill the pan only about ¾ of the way up.

6. Seal the pot, and cook on low pressure for 50 minutes.

7. Release the pressure with a quick release. The top of the pancake should be pale and sticky, but set, and it should be pulling away from the sides of the pan.

8. Carefully turn the pancake out onto a plate and serve. with fresh fruit or sliced figs, if desired.

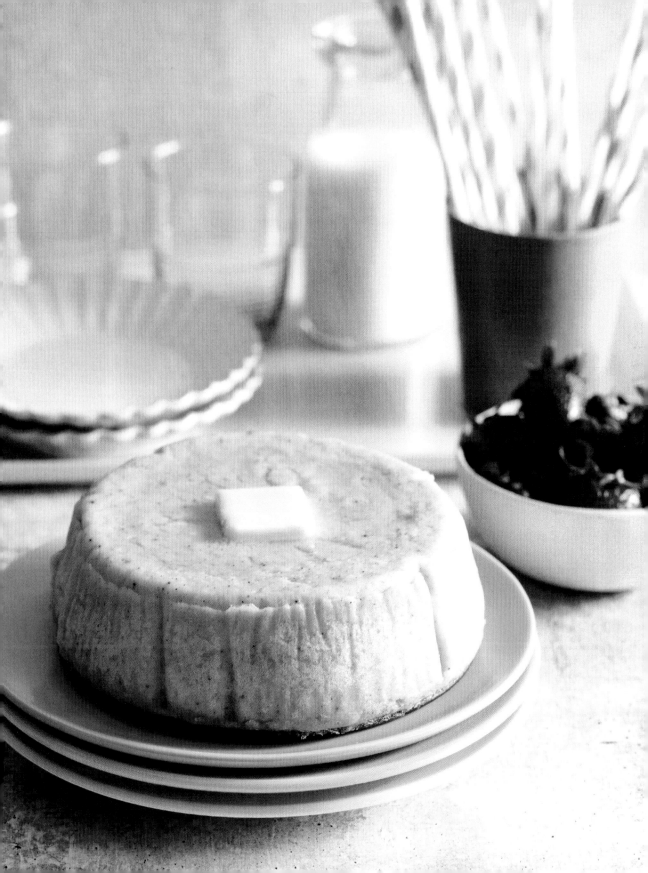

Breakfast Casserole for a Crowd

Here's proof that the Instant Pot isn't just for beans and soups: This delectable casserole is perfect for feeding your entire family or serving at your next brunch gathering. With pesto, spinach, and asparagus, you get green eggs, and when you add prosciutto you've got the time-tested kid favorite of green eggs and ham!

SERVES 6 TO 8

2 tablespoons extra virgin olive oil

1 large onion, minced

1 teaspoon sea salt

1½ cups very small broccoli florets

2 cups baby spinach

1 cup chopped asparagus

½ cup finely sliced prosciutto (optional)

6 large omega-3 eggs

½ cup coconut or almond milk

2 tablespoons basil pesto (store bought or homemade)

¼ cup grated Parmigiano-Reggiano or nutritional yeast (optional)

1. Set your Instant Pot to sauté, and heat the oil, onion, and salt. Cook for 2 to 3 minutes, until the onion begin to soften.

2. Add the broccoli, spinach, and asparagus, and cook, stirring occasionally, until the vegetables are tender.

3. Transfer to a bowl, and mix in the prosciutto, if using.

4. In a separate bowl, whisk together the eggs, milk, pesto, and Parmigiano-Reggiano or nutritional yeast, if using, and set aside.

5. Grease an oven-proof casserole dish or baking dish that'll fit inside your Instant Pot (you can also line it with parchment if you're *really* worried about sticking).

6. Transfer the vegetable mixture to the casserole dish, and top with the egg mixture.

7. Pour 1½ cups of water into the Instant Pot and set the metal trivet inside. Carefully set the casserole dish on the trivet.

8. Lock the lid, and cook on high pressure for 20 minutes.

9. Release the pressure with a quick release, and carefully remove the dish from the pot. Transfer onto a plate before serving.

Green Banana Bread

This gut-friendly twist on banana bread is so satisfying, you'll never go back to your old recipes that required you to wait for your bananas to turn into brown, overripe mush! Green bananas are an excellent source of resistant starch, making this bread a healthy way to start your day. Serve a slice on its own or topped with organic, full-fat cream cheese or goat's milk butter.

SERVES 6 TO 8

4 green bananas, broken up into chunks

1½ cups monk fruit sweetener

2 large omega-3 eggs

1 teaspoon pure banana extract (optional)

1 teaspoon pure vanilla extract

1¼ cups almond flour*

½ teaspoon cinnamon

½ teaspoon sea salt

1 teaspoon baking soda

½ cup bittersweet chocolate chips

½ cup toasted walnuts

Full fat cream cheese or goat's milk butter (optional)

*If you can find green banana flour, it's a great option here, too.

1. In a food processor fitted with an S-blade, add the green bananas and sweetener and blend until a very smooth purée is formed.

2. Add the eggs, the banana extract, if using, and the vanilla extract and pulse until smooth, and set aside.

3. In a large bowl, whisk together the almond flour, cinnamon, salt, and baking soda.

4. Fold the wet ingredients into the dry ingredients, and mix in the chocolate chips and toasted walnuts.

5. Grease a cake pan that fits into your Instant Pot (I like a 6- or 7-inch springform pan) and line it with parchment.

6. Pour the batter into the pan, and cover with foil.

7. Pour 1½ cups of water into the bottom of your Instant Pot, add the trivet, and carefully add the pan to the pot.

8. Lock the lid and cook on high pressure for 40 minutes.

9. Release the pressure with a quick release, and carefully remove the pan from the pot. It will look a little spongy, but that's okay—it's a super moist cake.

10. Let cool before turning out, then slice and top as desired.

French Toast, Two Ways

Kristine Anderson Wylie of "Lectin-Free Gourmet" says that French toast has always been a favorite dish in her family, so she was determined to make a Plant Paradox–friendly version that everyone could enjoy together. In the two recipes that follow, she offers both a sweet and a savory take on this breakfast classic. She makes her own baguette to use as the base, but you can use any lectin-free bread you happen to have on hand.

Classic French Toast Bake

SERVES 8

Coconut oil, for greasing the pan

1 Quick Baguette (page 185), or about 8 ounces of other lectin-free bread

¼ cup melted French or Italian butter, or avocado oil

¼ cup firmly-packed brown Swerve

1 tablespoon Lakanto Maple Flavored Syrup

3 large omega-3 eggs

1 cup heavy cream or coconut cream

2 teaspoons vanilla extract

2 teaspoons cinnamon

¼ teaspoon sea salt

In season fruit, fresh mint, and whipped coconut cream, to serve

1. Preheat the oven to 350°F. Grease a 9-inch pie dish with coconut oil, and set aside.

2. Cube the bread into bite-size pieces, and place in the prepared pie dish.

3. In a small saucepan over medium heat, add the butter or oil, Swerve, and syrup, and stir until bubbly and well combined, then set aside to cool.

4. In a high-speed blender, combine the eggs, cream, vanilla extract, cinnamon, and salt, and blend until smooth.

5. When the butter mixture is cool, add to the blender with the eggs and blitz to combine.

6. Pour the custard mixture over the bread, making sure it is distributed evenly.

7. Bake for 40 to 45 minutes, until the bread cubes are a dark golden brown and the custard has set.

8. Remove from the oven, and let stand for 5 minutes before serving.

9. Serve with the fruit, mint, and whipped coconut cream, or let everyone in the family choose their own toppings.

Savory Bánh Mì French Toast Bake

SERVES 8

Coconut oil, for greasing the pan

1 Quick Baguette (page 185), or about 8 ounces of other lectin-free bread

3 large pastured or omega-3 eggs

1 cup heavy cream or coconut cream

¼ cup melted French or Italian butter, or avocado oil

2 tablespoons minced lemongrass

1 tablespoon coconut aminos

1 tablespoon fish sauce

1 tablespoon Swerve

½ teaspoon five spice powder

2 cloves garlic, minced

2 green onions, sliced, white and green parts

Traditional Báhn Mi Pickled Vegetables, to serve (recipe follows)

Mint, cilantro, basil, watercress, and lime wedges, to serve

MAKES 3 CUPS PICKLED VEGETABLES

1 cup water

¼ cup Swerve

¼ cup fish sauce

¼ cup lime juice

¼ cup white wine vinegar

2 cloves garlic, minced

¼ teaspoon Sriracha, plus more to taste

1 cup thinly sliced carrots

1 cup thinly sliced daikon radish

1 small red onion, thinly sliced

1. Preheat the oven to 350°F. Grease a 9-inch pie dish with coconut oil, and set aside.

2. Cube the bread into bite-size pieces and arrange in the prepared pie dish.

3. In a high-speed blender, combine the eggs, cream, butter or oil, lemongrass, coconut aminos, fish sauce, Swerve, five spice powder, and garlic.

4. Pour the custard over the bread cubes, making sure it is distributed evenly. Sprinkle the green onions over the top.

5. Bake for 40 to 45 minutes, until the bread cubes are a dark golden brown and the custard has set.

6. Remove from the oven, and let stand for 5 minutes before serving.

7. Serve with the pickled vegetables, mint, cilantro, basil, watercress, and lime wedges, or let everyone in the family do their own toppings.

TRADITIONAL BÁNH MI PICKLED VEGETABLES

1. In a medium bowl, combine the water, Swerve, fish sauce, lime juice, vinegar, garlic, and Sriracha.

2. Add the carrots, radishes, and onion.

3. Let the vegetables marinate for at least 20 minutes before serving. Store leftovers in an airtight container in the fridge for up to a week

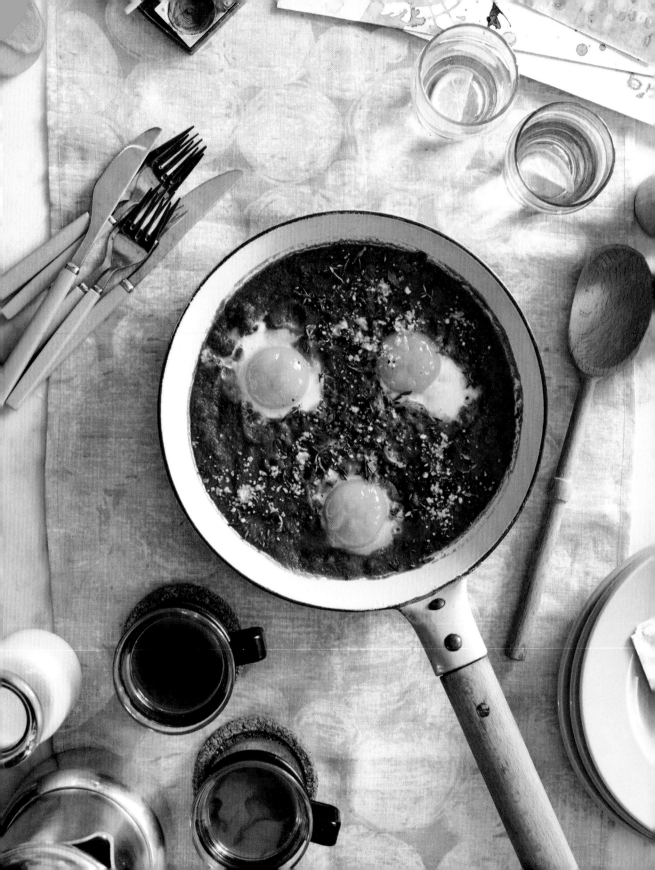

Shakshuka

This Middle Eastern egg dish has become increasingly popular in recent years—especially on brunch menus. Save yourself the money (and the effort of actually getting out of your pjs) and make this delicious dish at home! I like to add cauliflower rice and mushrooms to my Shakshuka for texture, flavor, and extra nutritional heft. A little bit of cocoa powder imbues the flavorful tomato sauce with some earthy notes, and a touch of grated Parmigiano-Reggiano at the end delivers a welcome punch of umami.

SERVES 4 TO 6

¼ cup extra-virgin olive oil

1 red onion, finely chopped

4 cloves garlic, minced

1 cup finely minced mushrooms

2 cups cauliflower rice

2 tablespoons minced fresh rosemary

1 tablespoon minced fresh thyme

1 teaspoon sea salt

½ teaspoon paprika

½ teaspoon dried basil

¼ teaspoon cinnamon

4 cups peeled, seeded, and chopped Italian canned tomatoes

1 tablespoon natural cocoa powder

8 large omega-3 eggs

Grated Parmigiano-Reggiano, for serving (optional)

1. Set your Instant Pot to sauté, and add the oil and onion and cook, stirring occasionally, until the onion is tender.

2. Add the garlic, mushrooms, cauliflower rice, rosemary, thyme, salt, paprika, basil, and cinnamon and continue to sauté until all the vegetables are tender and the mixture is very fragrant (it should start to smell a little like meat sauce).

3. Then add the tomatoes and cocoa powder and stir. Lock the lid, and cook on high pressure for 25 minutes.

4. Release the pressure with a quick release, and using an immersion blender*, puree the tomato sauce.

5. Carefuly crack the eggs into the blended sauce—avoid breaking the yolks. Lock the lid on your Instant Pot, and cook on low pressure for 1 minute.

6. Release the pressure with a quick release, and serve. Garnish with the Parmigiano-Reggiano, if using. It's great as is, or over cauliflower rice.

*You can also transfer your sauce to a high-speed blender to purée, but the immersion blender is much easier, if you've got one.

Cranberry-Orange Breakfast Bread

This sweet, tangy bread is just the thing with a cup of coffee in the morning—or the afternoon! If you're lucky enough to find fresh organic or local cranberries (which can be difficult) buy a few bags in the month of November and freeze them to enjoy the tart, bright zing of cranberries in this delicious bread all year long.

100% olive oil or avocado oil cooking spray

⅓ cup monk fruit sweetener or granulated Swerve

1 cup fresh or frozen cranberries

Finely grated zest of 1 large orange

4 large omega-3 eggs

1 teaspoon vanilla extract

1 teaspoon almond extract

⅓ cup coconut milk

¼ cup avocado oil

2¼ cups blanched almond flour

¾ teaspoon baking soda

¼ teaspoon sea salt

1. Preheat the oven to 350°F. Line a 8 x 4-inch loaf pan with parchment and spray with oil, and set aside.

2. In a food processor fitted with an S-blade, pulse the sweetener, cranberries, and orange zest until the cranberries are broken into small chunks, and set aside.

3. In a large bowl, whisk together the eggs, vanilla and almond extracts, coconut milk, and avocado oil.

4. In a separate bowl, combine the almond flour, baking soda, salt, and cranberry mixture.

5. Fold the flour mixture into the wet mixture until well combined.

6. Transfer to the prepared loaf pan and bake for 40 to 50 minutes, until a toothpick inserted into the middle of the loaf comes out clean.

7. Let cool completely before serving.

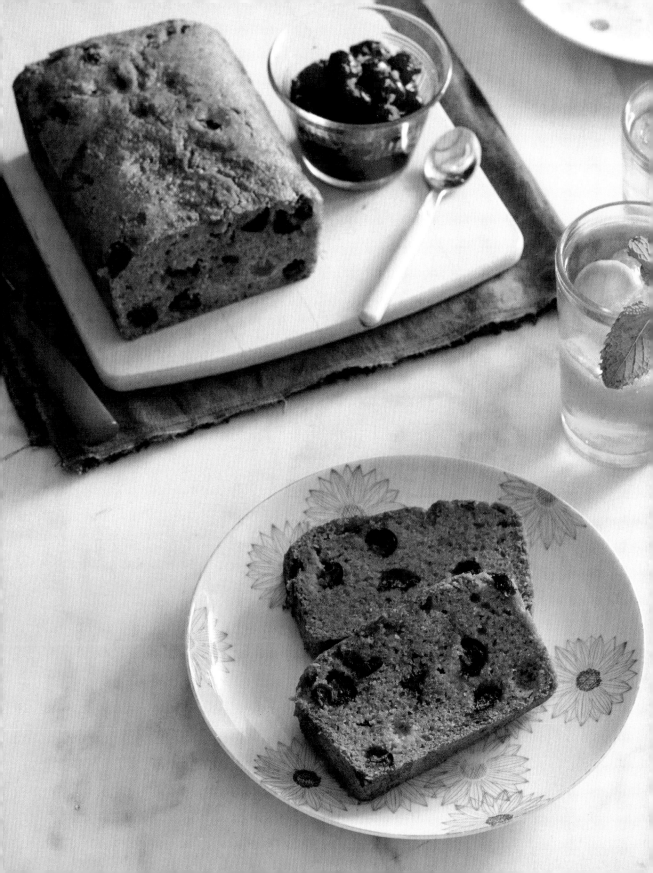

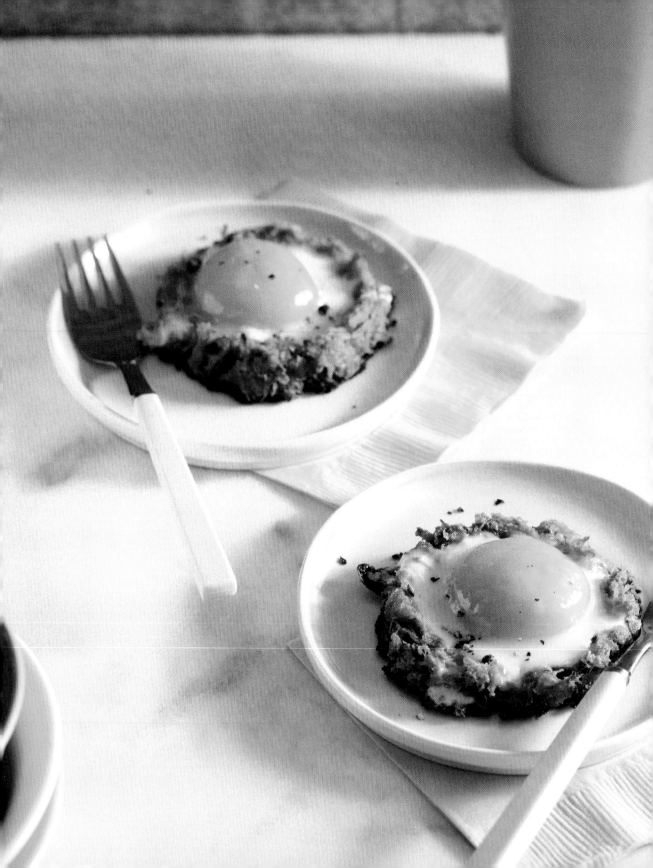

Sweet Potato Egg Nests

Kids love these little egg-filled "birds nests," which also make an elegant breakfast or brunch option for grown ups. And everyone will benefit from starting off their day with the perfect combination of fat, protein, and veggies. If your pesto turns brown while the nests are cooking in the oven, don't worry—they will still taste delicious! If you'd like, you can spoon a little fresh pesto on top for color before serving.

SERVES 6

100% olive oil or avocado oil cooking spray (used twice)

1½ cups shredded sweet potatoes

1½ cups broccoli slaw

1 teaspoon sea salt

4 tablespoons tapioca starch, more as needed

1 teaspoon black pepper

1 teaspoon garlic powder

7 large omega-3 eggs

¼ cup basil pesto (optional)

¼ cup extra-virgin olive oil

1. Preheat the oven to 375°F. Line a sheet tray with a Silpat or parchment, and spray with oil, and set aside.

2. In a large bowl, combine the sweet potatoes, broccoli slaw, and salt and let sit for 5 to 10 minutes to draw out the moisture.

3. Pat the vegetable mixture dry, then transfer to a bowl. Add the tapioca starch, pepper, garlic powder, and 1 egg, and stir to combine.

4. Check the consistency of the mixture—it should be somewhat dry, but cohesive enough to hold together when formed into patties or balls.

5. Divide the mixture into 6 equal-size mounds on the prepared sheet tray, shaping them into "nests" with a hollow in the center. Spray the nests with cooking spray.

6. Place in the oven and bake for 15 to 20 minutes, until tender.

7. Remove from the oven and brush with the basil pesto, if using.

8. Crack 1 egg into each of the hollows in the "nests" and return to the oven.

9. Bake an additional 5 to 15 minutes, depending on how you like your eggs cooked.

10. Remove from the oven, drizzle with olive oil, and serve.

chapter six

Single-Pan Suppers

Skillet "Pizza"

I have yet to meet a kid who doesn't love pizza, but traditional wheat crusts and tomato sauce aren't good for anyone. With Dr. G's Tomato Sauce and a satisfyingly chewy cauliflower crust that can be made and frozen ahead of time, this skillet pizza transforms an old favorite into a brand-new kid pleaser.

MAKES 1 (12-INCH) PIE

FOR THE CRUST:

100% olive oil cooking spray

1 head cauliflower or 1 pound cauliflower rice

¾ cup grated Parmigiano-Reggiano

1½ teaspoons garlic powder

1½ teaspoons onion powder

¼ cup almond flour

2 tablespoons tapioca flour

1 4-oz ball mozzarella (Italian or Buffalo), shredded

1½ large omega-3 eggs*

*To measure half an egg, scramble a whole egg, and use half of it (by weight).

1. Preheat the oven to 425°F. (If making the pizza immediately, leave the oven on after baking the crust while you put together the toppings.)

2. Spray a 12-inch oven-safe skillet with oil and line the bottom with parchment, and set aside.

3. In the bowl of a food processor fitted with an S-blade, add the cauliflower and pulse until a fine powder is formed. Transfer to a clean dishcloth, and twist the cloth to wring out all the moisture.

4. In a large bowl, add the cauliflower, Parmigiano-Reggiano, garlic and onion powders, almond and tapioca flours, mozzarella, and eggs and mix well to combine.

5. Place the mixture into the prepared skillet and pat down, making sure to get the dough up the sides of the skillet.

6. Place the skillet in the oven and bake for 20 to 25 minutes, until golden brown, then remove from the oven and fill according to the instructions on the following page.

Note: You can also make the crust ahead of time in a cake pan, and freeze it once it's cooled. When you're ready, go ahead and follow the "for the pizza" steps on the next page, and cook right in the frozen crust. It's always good to have a crust on hand for those busy nights!

¼ cup extra-virgin olive oil

1 cup diced mushrooms

1 onion, minced

4 cloves garlic, minced

2 cups finely minced bitter greens (kale, mustard greens, chard, or spinach)

1 teaspoon fine sea salt

1 teaspoon dried oregano

½ teaspoon sweet paprika

½ teaspoon freshly ground black pepper

½ teaspoon powdered garlic

1 prepared crust, (recipe above)

1 cup shredded buffalo mozzarella or creamy Garlic and Chive "Cheese" Spread (page 173)

1½ cups Dr. G's Tomato Sauce (page 221) or basil pesto

1. Preheat the oven to 425ºF.

2. In a large skillet over medium high, heat the oil. Add the mushrooms, onion, and garlic, and cook, stirring occasionally, until the onion is translucent and the mushrooms are tender.

3. Add the bitter greens, salt, oregano, paprika, black pepper, and garlic powder, and cook until the greens are wilted and the whole mixture is very fragrant. Remove from the heat and set aside.

4. To assemble the pizza, add a thin layer of the buffalo mozzarella to the bottom of the crust, followed by half the bitter greens mixture.

5. Add a bit more cheese, the tomato sauce, then top with the remaining greens mixture, and buffalo mozzarella.

6. Place in the oven, and bake for 20 minutes, until warmed through and melty.

7. Slice carefully and serve, being aware that this pie does not hold its shape as well as a traditional pizza. (Bowls are a great option!)

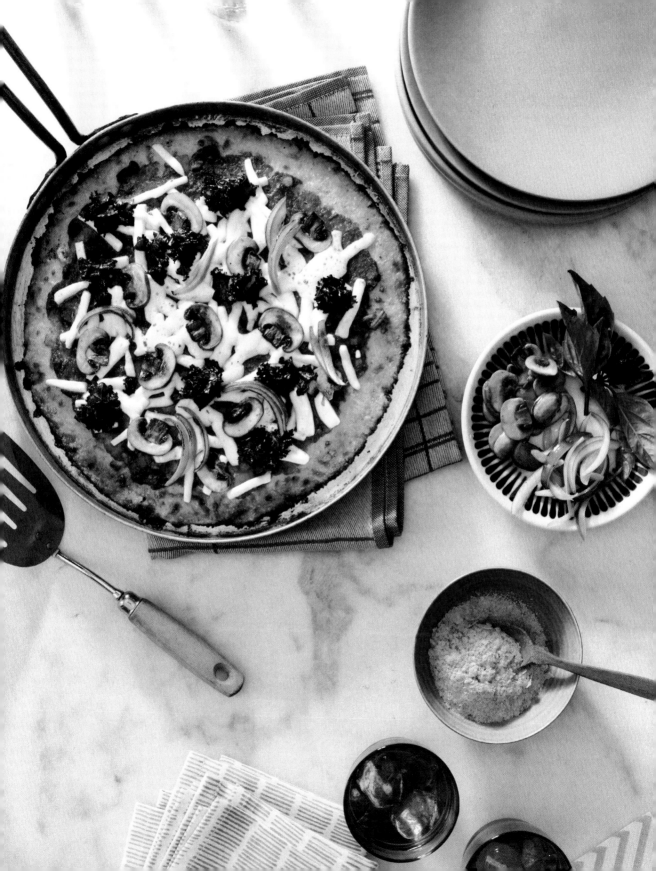

Pastured Chicken Nuggets

Some kids (and more than a few adults) seem to exist entirely on prepackaged and fast foods like chicken nuggets, but that's no diet for a growing child—or anyone else. My pastured chicken nuggets are just as crispy, tender, and delicious as the nuggets you're used to, and cooking with the Instant Pot ensures there will be gut-friendly ketchup for dipping on the side!

SERVES 4

100% olive oil cooking spray (for cooking in oven)

¼ cup extra-virgin olive oil

1 cup diced mushrooms

½ pound pasture-raised boneless chicken breast

1 teaspoon Old Bay Seasoning

1 tablespoon Dijon mustard

1 tablespoon minced fresh rosemary

½ cup tapioca starch

¼ cup psyllium husk flakes

¼ cup almond flour

1 large omega-3 egg

Tangy Ranch Dressing/Dip (page 219), for serving

Lectin-Light Ketchup (page 220), for serving

1 teaspoon sea salt after cooking

1. Line a rimmed baking sheet with parchment, and set aside.

2. Heat a large skillet over medium high. Add the oil and mushrooms and sauté until the mushrooms are browned and tender. Remove from the heat and let cool to room temperature.

3. In the bowl of a food processor fitted with an S-blade, pulse together the chicken breast, Old Bay, mustard, and rosemary until finely chopped.

4. Add the mushroom mixture along with 2 tablespoons of the tapioca starch, and pulse until a smooth paste is formed. You should be able to form "nuggets" with your hands. If not, add more tapioca starch, a bit at a time, until the mixture binds together.

5. Shape the chicken mixture into nuggets, and space evenly on the prepared baking sheet.

6. Freeze for 15 to 20 minutes, until fairly solid, and easy to handle.

7. Meanwhile, in a small bowl, combine the remaining tapioca starch, the psyllium husk, and almond flour.

8. In a separate bowl, beat the egg.

9. When the nuggets are semi-frozen, dip each in the egg mixture, then in the tapioca starch mixture, coating evenly, and set aside.

10. Cook the nuggets using one of the two methods below, or return to the baking sheet and freeze. Once frozen solid, you can transfer them to a zip-top bag for more convenient storage.

TO COOK IN THE OVEN:

1. Spray a baking sheet with oil, and place in a cold oven. Preheat the oven (and baking sheet) to 425ºF.

2. When hot, remove the baking sheet and spray with an additional coating of olive oil. Transfer the nuggets to the baking sheet, spreading into a single layer, and spray the tops with olive oil.

3. Bake for 8 to 10 minutes, then flip, and bake for another 4 to 5 minutes, until a thermometer inserted into the thickest nugget reaches 165ºF. Sprinkle with the salt after cooking.

4. Serve with the ranch dressing, ketchup, and a great big green salad.

TO COOK IN AN AIR FRYER:

1. Preheat the air fryer to 380ºF.

2. Spray the fryer basket with olive oil, and arrange the nuggets in a single layer in the basket. You may need to cook in batches.

3. Cook for 5 to 6 minutes, then flip the nuggets and cook for an additional 5 to 6 minutes. Sprinkle with the salt after cooking.

4. Serve with the ranch dressing, ketchup, and a great big green salad.

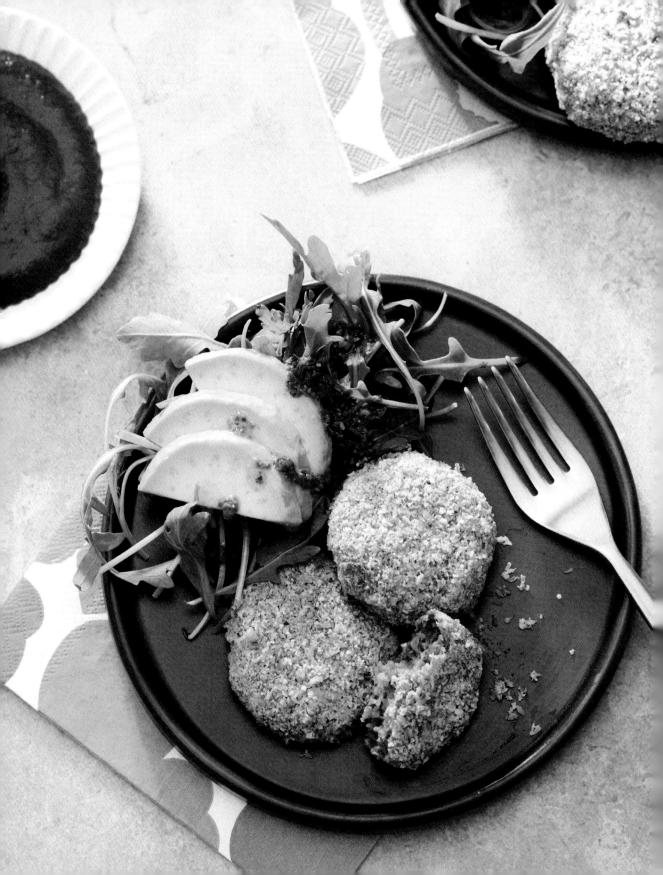

Quorn "Chicken" Nuggets

If you're unfamiliar with Quorn, the vegetarian protein that's widely available in supermarkets, I recommend giving this recipe a try. With the sweet potato and egg acting as binders, these nuggets hold their shape well and are absolutely delicious. For families who are looking to cut down on animal protein, Quorn is a great choice and these nuggets will soon become a go-to staple. I recommend making a double batch and stashing some in the freezer!

SERVES 4

100% olive oil cooking spray (for cooking in oven)

1 tablespoon extra-virgin olive oil

1 cup diced mushrooms

½ cup minced onions

1 tablespoon Old Bay Seasoning

1 tablespoon minced fresh rosemary

1 bag Quorn grounds, thawed

1 small sweet potato, baked, skin removed, mashed (about ½ cup)

½ cup tapioca starch

¼ cup psyllium husk flakes

¼ cup almond flour

1 large omega-3 egg

1 teaspoon sea salt

Tangy Ranch Dressing/Dip (page 219), for serving

Lectin-Light Ketchup (page 220), for serving

1. Line a rimmed baking sheet with parchment, and set aside.

2. Heat a large skillet over medium high. Add the oil, mushrooms, and onions and sauté until the onions are translucent and the mushrooms are brown and tender. Add the Old Bay seasoning and rosemary and continue to sauté until very fragrant.

3. Transfer the mixture to the work bowl of a food processor fitted with an S-blade, and pulse together the mushroom, onion and seasoning mixture, the Quorn, and the sweet potato until well combined. The mixture should be a little chunky.

4. Transfer to a bowl and add 2 tablespoons of tapioca starch. Stir to combine. You should be able to form "nuggets" with your hands. If not, add more tapioca starch, a teaspoon at a time, until the nuggets bind together.

5. Shape the mixture into nuggets, about 1 to 2 tablespoons each, and space evenly on the prepared baking sheet.

6. Freeze for 15 to 20 minutes, until fairly solid and easy to handle.

7. Meanwhile, in a small bowl, combine the remaining tapioca starch, the psyllium husk, and almond flour.

8. In a separate bowl, beat the egg.

9. When the nuggets are semi-frozen, dip each in the egg mixture, then in the tapioca starch mixture, coating evenly, and set aside.

10. Cook using one of the two methods below, or return to the baking sheet and freeze. Once frozen solid, you can transfer them to a zip-top bag for more convenient storage.

TO COOK IN THE OVEN:

1. Spray a baking sheet with oil, and place in a cold oven. Preheat the oven (and baking sheet) to 425°F.

2. When the baking sheet is hot, spray with an additional coating of oil. Transfer the nuggets to the baking sheet, spreading into a single layer, and spray the tops with olive oil.

3. Bake for 8 to 10 minutes, then flip, and bake for another 4 to 5 minutes, until a thermometer inserted into the thickest nugget reaches 165°F. Sprinkle with the salt after cooking.

4. Serve with the ranch dressing, ketchup, and a great big green salad.

TO COOK IN AN AIR FRYER:

1. Preheat the air fryer to 380°F.

2. Spray the fryer basket with olive oil, and arrange the nuggets in a single layer in the basket. You may need to cook in batches.

3. Cook for 5 to 6 minutes, then flip the nuggets and cook for an additional 5 to 6 minutes. Sprinkle with the salt after cooking.

4. Serve with the ranch dressing, ketchup, and a great big green salad.

Beef and (Mostly) Broccoli

I love beef and broccoli as much as the next guy, so I wanted to make over one of my favorite Chinese menu take-out dishes so that I could still enjoy it in a healthy way. And here's the best part: This recipe is super easy and fast to make, offers a ton of flavor, and is a guaranteed crowd pleaser. Be sure to purchase 100 percent grass-fed (or grass-fed and finished) beef for this tasty dinner. For easier slicing against the grain, place the meat in the freezer for 15 to 20 minutes to firm it up.

SERVES 4 TO 6

Avocado oil cooking spray

1 pound grass-fed flank steak, cut against the grain into thin slices (you can also use sliced tempeh, jackfruit, or a mixture of any of the three)

4 to 5 cloves garlic, finely minced

2 tablespoons fresh minced ginger

1 tablespoon monk fruit sweetener or local honey

2 tablespoons toasted sesame oil

2 tablespoons unsweetened rice wine vinegar

½ cup coconut aminos

1 bunch green onions, finely sliced, whites and greens separated

1 large yellow onion, thinly sliced

6 cups broccoli florets

1 tablespoon toasted sesame seeds

1. Preheat the oven to 425°F. Lightly spray a rimmed baking sheet with oil, and set aside.

2. In a zip-top bag, combine the steak, garlic, ginger, sweetener, sesame oil, vinegar, coconut aminos, and the whites of the green onions. Let marinate for 20 to 25 minutes.

3. In a large bowl, add the yellow onion and broccoli, and pour the steak mixture over the broccoli mixture. Toss to combine well, then transfer to the prepared baking sheet.

4. Bake for 15 to 20 minutes, until the steak has reached your desired level of doneness and the broccoli is tender.

5. Before serving, toss with the sesame seeds and the green parts of the green onions.

Serving Suggestion: Serve over steamed cauliflower rice, pressure-cooked basmati rice, or millet.

Cauliflower Broccoli Nuggets

Want to get your kids to eat more veggies? Put them in nugget form and they're bound to gobble them up. These deceptively healthy bites are packed with cruciferous vegetables and protein, making them a wonderfully easy and transportable whole-meal option for smaller kids. If your little ones are sensitive to spice, you may want to omit the Old Bay (though I personally love the flavor it adds!)

SERVES 4

100% olive oil cooking spray (for cooking in oven)

1½ cups broccoli florets, steamed until very tender

1½ cups cauliflower florets, steamed until very tender

2 tablespoons basil pesto (homemade or store bought)

½ cup shredded Parmigiano-Reggiano or nutritional yeast

1 cup ground flaxseed

1 tablespoon Old Bay Seasoning

½ cup tapioca starch

¼ cup psyllium husk flakes

¼ cup almond flour

1 to 2 large omega-3 eggs*

1 teaspoon sea salt

Tangy Ranch Dressing/Dip (page 219), for serving

Lectin-Light Ketchup (page 220), for serving

*To make this recipe vegan, omit the eggs, and brush nuggets in a light coating of Dijon before serving.

1. Line a rimmed baking sheet with parchment, and set aside.

2. In the work bowl of a food processor fitted with an S-blade, add the broccoli and cauliflower, and pulse until smooth.

3. Add the pesto, Parmigiano-Reggiano, ¾ cup flaxseed, the Old Bay, 2 tablespoons tapioca starch, and 1 tablespoon psyllium husk flakes and continue to pulse until smooth.

4. Let rest in the processor for 5 minutes. This should give the mixture time to stiffen. Mixture should form easily into nuggets—if too loose, add more tapioca starch, 1 teaspoon at a time, until stiff enough.

5. Using 2 spoons or a spring-loaded ice cream scoop, shape the mixture into 1 to 2 tablespoon-size "nuggets" and space evenly on the prepared baking sheet.

6. Freeze for 15 to 20 minutes, until fairly solid, and easy to handle.

7. Meanwhile, in a small bowl, combine the remaining tapioca starch, psyllium husk flakes, and almond flour.

8. In a separate bowl, beat the egg.

9. When the nuggets are semi-frozen, dip each in the egg mixture, then in the tapioca starch mixture, coating evenly, and set aside.

10. Cook using one of the two methods below, or return to the baking sheet to freeze. Once frozen solid, you can transfer them to a zip-top bag for more convenient storage.

You can store these for 2–3 months in the freezer.

TO COOK IN THE OVEN:

1. Spray a baking sheet with oil, and place in a cold oven. Preheat the oven (and baking sheet) to 425ºF.

2. When hot, spray the baking sheet with an additional coating of oil. Transfer the nuggets to the baking sheet, spreading into a single layer. Spray the nugget tops with olive oil.

3. Bake for 8 to 10 minutes, then flip, and bake for another 4 to 5 minutes, until heated through. Sprinkle with the salt after cooking.

4. Serve with the ranch dressing, ketchup, and a great big green salad.

TO COOK IN AN AIR FRYER:

1. Preheat the air fryer to 380ºF.

2. Spray the fryer basket with olive oil, and arrange the nuggets in a single layer in the basket. You may need to cook in batches.

3. Cook for 5 to 6 minutes, then flip the nuggets and cook for an additional 5 to 6 minutes. Sprinkle with the salt after cooking.

4. Serve with the ranch dressing, ketchup, and a great big green salad.

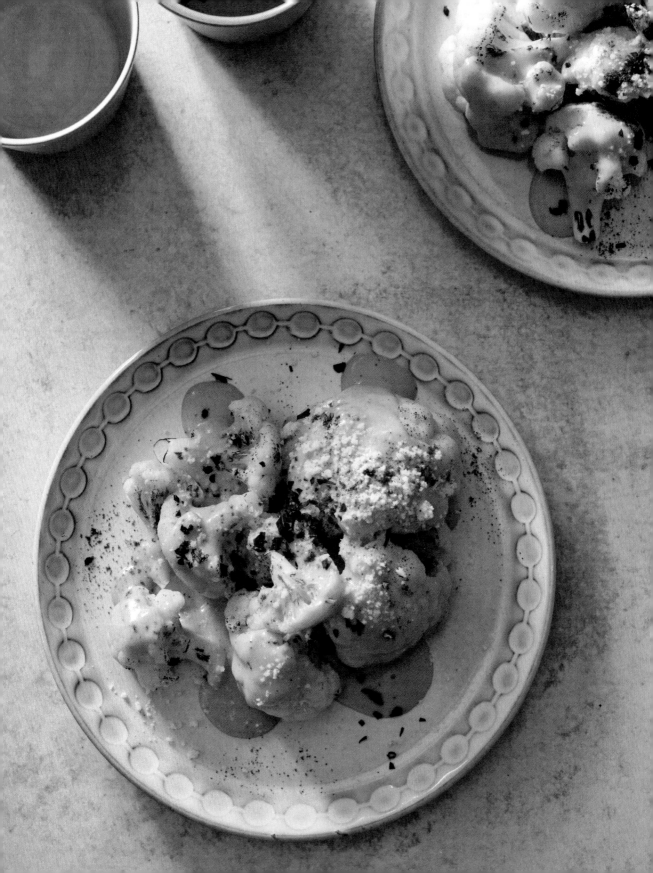

Cauliflower "Mac" and Cheese

Perfect on its own or with my BBQ Pulled Pork (page 145), this cauliflower "mac" and cheese is a play on one of the most popular American side dishes ever created. Here cauliflower shines as it takes the place of macaroni noodles with aplomb. This is the perfect dish to convert your kids to the Plant Paradox!

SERVES 6 TO 8

100% olive oil cooking spray

1 large head cauliflower, cut into small florets and steamed until tender

2 tablespoons coconut oil

2 tablespoons tapioca flour

1½ cups coconut milk

1 tablespoon Dijon mustard

½ teaspoon garlic powder

½ teaspoon smoked paprika

1 teaspoon sea salt or to taste

1¼ cups grated goat's milk Cheddar

¼ cup grated Parmigiano-Reggiano

To make this mac and cheese vegan, use 1 cup nutritional yeast instead of the cheeses.

1. Preheat the oven to 350°F. Spray an 8 x 8-inch baking dish with oil, and add the steamed cauliflower, and set aside.

2. In a large saucepan, heat the coconut oil. Add the tapioca flour and cook over low heat, stirring frequently, until golden brown.

3. Add the coconut milk, mustard, garlic powder, paprika, and salt, and continue to whisk for 3 to 5 minutes until the sauce begins to thicken.

4. Add the Cheddar to the sauce and continually whisk to combine.

5. Pour the cheese sauce over the cauliflower, and sprinkle with the Parmigiano-Reggiano.

6. Bake for 20 to 25 minutes, until bubbly and crispy on top.

Pistachio Chicken Croquettes with Honey-Mustard Sauce

Unlike traditional chicken nuggets, these pistachio-crusted croquettes from Claudia Curini of "Creative in My Kitchen" are delicious both hot and cold—meaning they're great for dinner, *and* as a lunch box option the next day. The "honey" mustard sauce not only pairs well with these croquettes (or any of the nugget recipes in this book), but also makes a great sandwich spread.

SERVES 4 TO 6

FOR THE CROQUETTES:

½ cup minced fresh parsley

¼ cup roughly chopped onion

¼ cup roughly chopped celery

½ cup tightly-packed fresh spinach leaves

2 cups cooked, shredded pasture-raised chicken

⅓ cup grated Parmigiano-Reggiano

3 tablespoons extra-virgin olive oil

¾ teaspoon sea salt

½ teaspoon freshly ground black pepper

¾ cup finely minced shelled pistachios (the consistency of breadcrumbs)

1. Preheat the oven to 450°F, and set the rack in the middle of your oven. Line a sheet tray with parchment, and set aside.

2. To make the croquettes, in the bowl of a food processor fitted with an S-blade, pulse the parsley, onion, celery, and spinach, until finely chopped.

3. Add the chicken and Parmigiano-Reggiano, and pulse until the mixture is well combined.

4. Then add the oil, salt, and pepper, and pulse until the mixture begins to form a paste that binds together and holds its shape easily.

5. Shape the mixture into small logs or balls, then roll each log in the pistachios.

6. Freeze the croquettes for 10 minutes.

7. Arrange the croquettes on the prepared sheet tray, place in the oven on the middle rack, and bake for 10 minutes.

½ cup avocado mayonnaise

1½ tablespoons Dijon mustard

Juice of ¼ lemon

2 teaspoons red wine vinegar

1 teaspoon yacon syrup

¼ teaspoon garlic powder

¼ teaspoon onion powder

¼ teaspoon curry powder

8. Make the sauce while the croquettes are baking. Combine all ingredients in a high-speed blender and blend until a smooth, well-combined sauce is formed. Set aside.

9. After 10 minutes, flip the croquettes and bake an additional 5 to 10 minutes, until golden brown and crispy to the touch.

10. Serve the croquettes warm or at room temperature with the honey-mustard sauce.

Autumn Sheet Pan Dinner

Sheet pan dinners are truly fantastic options for any meal, but especially on a busy weeknight. Throw together some ingredients on a sheet pan, roast them in the oven, and while dinner is prepping, you can set the table, help your kids with their homework, or just take a minute to relax with a glass of red wine. For a vegetarian option, swap out the turkey breast for a whole head of cauliflower. It makes for a show-stopping meal!

SERVES 4 WITH LEFTOVERS

1 3 to 4 pound bone-in, skin-on pastured or kosher turkey breast*

1½ teaspoons sea salt

2 small sweet potatoes, cut into ¼-inch slices

1 yellow onion, cut into bite-size chunks

4 cups Brussels sprouts, halved

½ cup extra-virgin olive oil

4 cloves garlic, minced

2 tablespoons fresh minced sage

1 tablespoon fresh minced thyme

1 teaspoon freshly ground black pepper

1 teaspoon dried poultry seasoning

To make vegetarian as pictured here, swap out the turkey breast for a whole head of cauliflower, and drizzled with olive oil before roasting.

1. Preheat the oven to 375°F.

2. Remove the turkey breast from the refrigerator, and sprinkle with about ½ teaspoon of the salt, and let sit at room temperature while the oven heats.

3. Pat the turkey dry with paper towels, and place on one side of a baking sheet, skin-side up.

4. Put the turkey in the oven and roast for 30 minutes.

5. Meanwhile, in a large bowl, combine the sweet potatoes, onion, and Brussels sprouts.

6. In another bowl, whisk together the oil, garlic, sage, thyme, pepper, and poultry seasoning, then pour over the vegetable mixture, and toss to combine.

7. Carefully transfer the vegetables to the baking sheet with the turkey, and roast for 15 minutes, then carefully toss the vegetables with a wooden spoon. Continue roasting for about 15 more minutes until the Brussels sprouts' leaves are crisp, the sweet potatoes are tender, the turkey is 165°F, and your whole house smells like Thanksgiving.

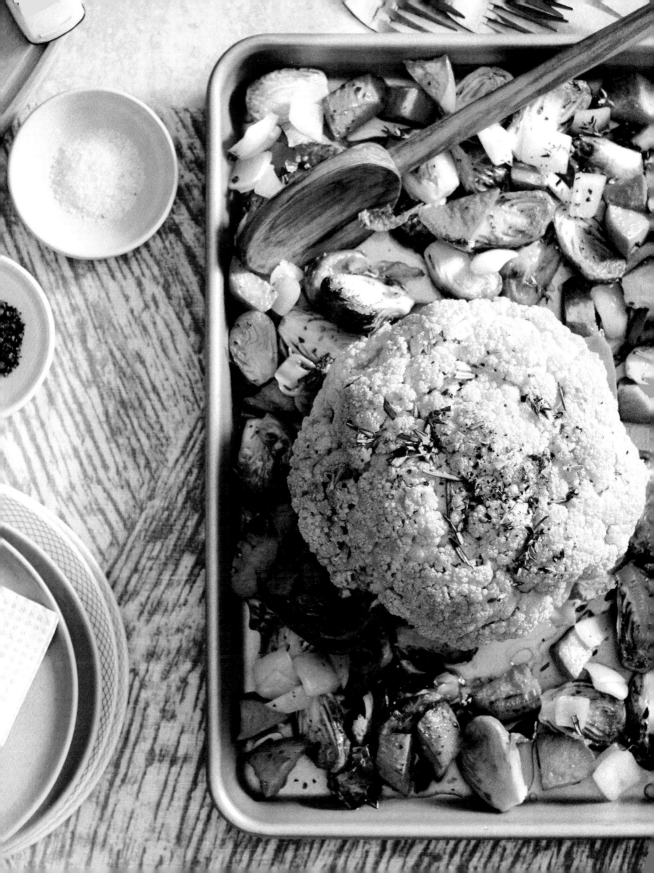

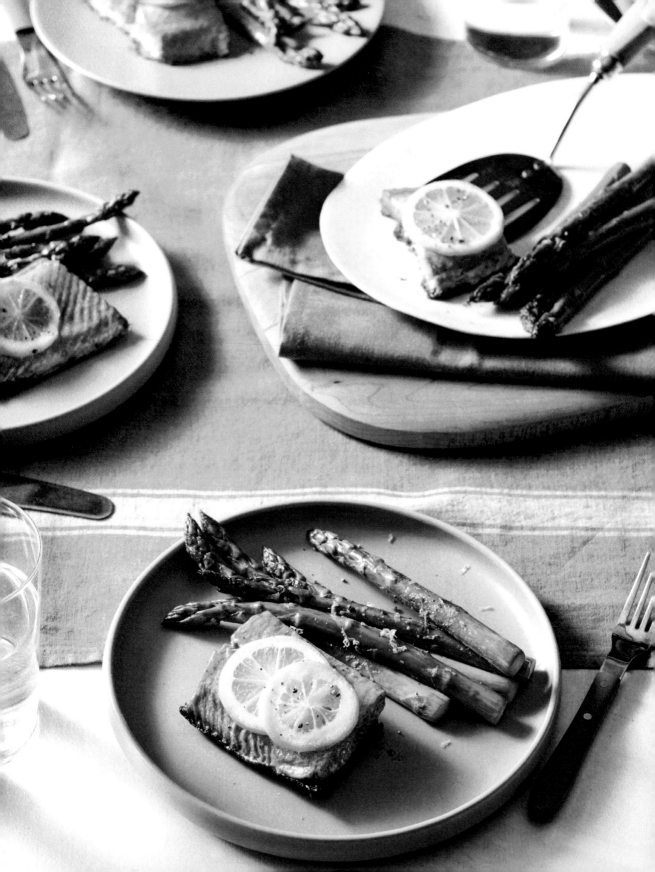

Lemony Salmon and Asparagus

Here is another perfect for weeknight sheet pan dinner. This one features omega-3- rich wild-caught and delicious asparagus. The dinner practically cooks itself and requires very little cleanup. What comes out of the oven is so flavorful and elegant, it feels as if you have somehow cheated on dinner prep!

SERVES 4

100% olive oil cooking spray

1½ teaspoons sea salt

½ teaspoon freshly ground black pepper

¼ teaspoon smoked paprika

⅛ teaspoon cinnamon

2 large lemons

1 pound wild caught salmon, cut into four 4-ounce fillets, skin on*

¼ cup extra-virgin olive oil

4 cloves garlic, minced

1 tablespoon fresh rosemary

1½ pounds asparagus, tough ends trimmed.

To make vegetarian, try using sliced tempeh or jackfruit in place of the salmon.

1. Preheat the oven to 350°F. Lightly spray a rimmed baking sheet with oil, and set aside.

2. In a small bowl, whisk together ½ teaspoon of the salt, the black pepper, paprika, and cinnamon.

3. Zest the lemons, and add the zest to the spice mixture.

4. Liberally sprinkle the mixture on the salmon, and place the salmon, skin side down, on the prepared baking sheet.

5. Slice 1 lemon, and lay the slices over the salmon.

6. In a small bowl, juice the remaining lemon, discarding the seeds, and add the olive oil, garlic, rosemary, and the remaining salt, and whisk to combine.

7. Place the prepared asparagus on the baking sheet along with the salmon, and pour the lemon sauce over the asparagus.

8. Bake for 15 to 20 minutes, until the salmon flakes easily with a fork.

9. Serve, and enjoy.

Sheet Pan Fajitas

This is a great dinner to prep in advance when you're planning to entertain—you can get your veggies ready to go and make the sauce a day ahead of time. Then, when it comes time for dinner, all you need to do is add your ingredients to a sheet pan and turn on the oven! Serve with fresh guacamole, Spicy Tomato Salsa (page 225), and a handful of cassava flour chips for a festive meal.

SERVES 4 TO 6

¼ cup extra-virgin olive oil plus extra for greasing baking sheet

1 pound thinly-sliced tempeh, flank steak, wild caught shrimp, or Quorn crumbles

2 red onions, thinly sliced

3 portobello mushroom caps, thinly sliced

3 cups broccoli florets

Stems from 1 bunch rainbow chard, sliced (save the leaves for something else, or use them as wraps for your fajitas)

1 small bunch (8 to 10 sprigs) cilantro

2 cloves garlic

1 lime, quartered

1½ teaspoons cumin

1½ teaspoons sea salt

1 teaspoon smoked paprika

Cassava tortillas (Siete brand), for serving

Spicy Tomato Salsa (page 225), for serving

Guacamole or avocado slices, for serving

Grated goat's milk cheddar, for serving

1. Preheat the oven to 425°F. Lightly grease a rimmed baking sheet with oil, and set aside.

2. In a large bowl, add the protein, onions, mushrooms, broccoli, and rainbow chard stems.

3. In your high-speed blender or the bowl of a food processor fitted with an S-blade, blend the oil, cilantro, garlic, lime, cumin, salt, and paprika until smooth.

4. Pour the sauce over the protein and vegetables, and toss to combine. This is a great place to get little ones involved!

5. Turn the whole mixture out onto the prepared baking sheet, and spread to one even layer.

6. Bake for 5 to 10 minutes, then toss, and bake an additional 5 to 10 minutes.

7. If you like a "charred" flavor, switch your oven to broil, and broil for 3 to 4 minutes, watching carefully so the vegetables don't burn.

8. Serve family-style with cassava tortillas, salsa, guacamole, and cheese.

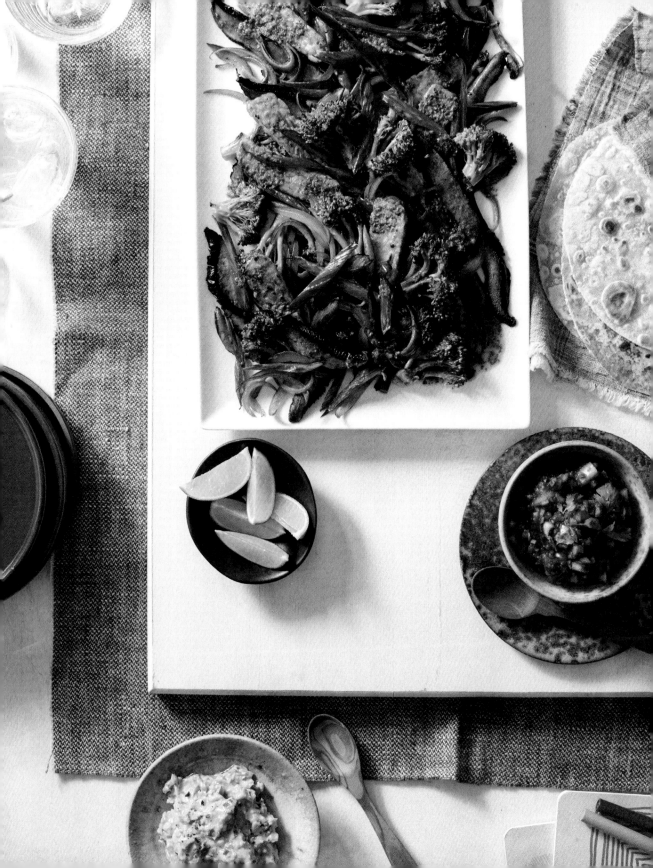

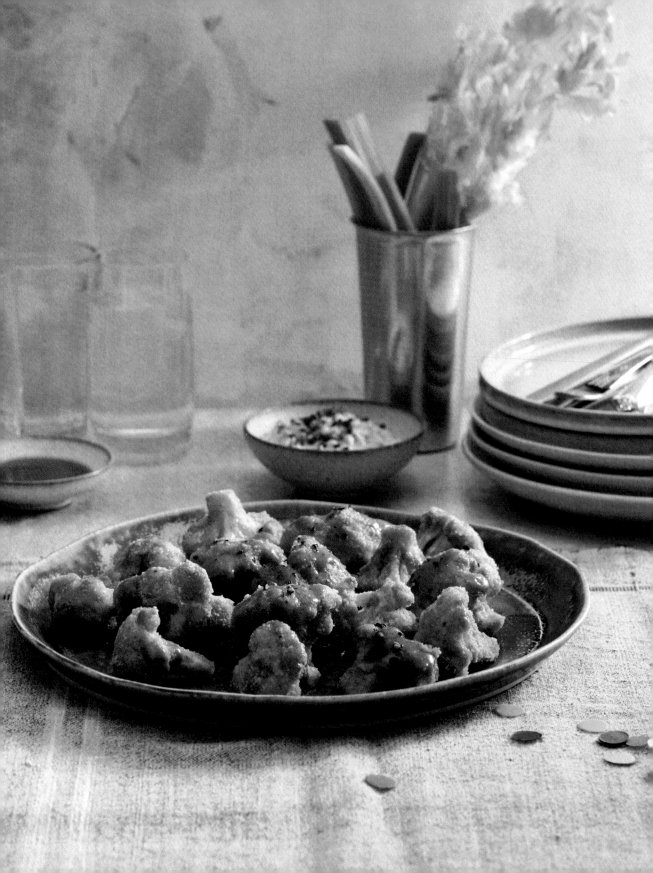

Not-Too-Spicy Buffalo "Wings"

You might not believe me when I say I prefer these "wings" to chicken wings, but it's true! Roasted cauliflower develops a satisfying, meaty texture, which pairs perfectly with a spicy homemade buffalo sauce. Pair the "wings" with a green salad for a complete meal, or serve them as an appetizer at your next party. Your guests will love them!

SERVES 4

FOR THE "WINGS":

¼ cup avocado oil or olive oil plus extra for spraying pan

1 cup almond flour

1 teaspoon garlic powder

1 teaspoon smoked paprika

½ teaspoon sea salt

1 large omega-3 egg or approved vegan egg substitute

3 cups cauliflower florets

FOR THE SAUCE:

¼ cup buffalo-style hot sauce (it's seeded, peeled, and fermented!)

¼ cup avocado oil or olive oil

1 teaspoon Dijon mustard

FOR THE DIP:

¼ cup Southern European blue cheese or nutritional yeast

1 cup coconut milk yogurt

½ teaspoon sea salt

1 tablespoon minced chives

Celery slices, for serving

1. Preheat the oven to 400°F. Spray a rimmed baking sheet with oil and set aside.

2. To make the "wings," in a large bowl, mix together the almond flour, garlic powder, paprika, and salt.

3. In a separate bowl, whisk the egg.

4. Dip the cauliflower florets in the egg mixture, then toss them in the almond flour mixture, coating evenly, and set aside.

5. Spread the prepared "wings" on the the baking sheet, and bake for 15 to 20 minutes, turning occasionally, until very crisp—cooking time will vary based on the size of your florets.

6. Meanwhile, to make the buffalo sauce, in a small bowl, combine the hot sauce, oil, and mustard, and set aside.

7. To make the dip, in a separate bowl, combine the blue cheese, yogurt, salt, and chives, and set aside.

8. When the cauliflower is crisp, remove from the oven and toss with the buffalo sauce before serving.

9. Serve with the blue cheese dip and celery slices on the side.

Tahini-Miso Tempeh

Red miso gives a truly satisfying umami taste to this vegan sheet pan dinner. Red miso ferments longer than white miso and thus has a deeper taste. Here, it infuses the tempeh a lot of flavor. Tahini serves as a mellowing agent to the miso, and also as a creamy element that makes this meatless dinner taste truly indulgent.

SERVES 4

Sesame oil or olive oil, for greasing pan

¼ cup tahini

¼ cup red miso paste

2 tablespoons coconut aminos

1 tablespoon balsamic vinegar

1 tablespoon monk fruit sweetener

1 pound tempeh, cut into bite-size cubes

1 pound quartered Brussels sprouts

1 yellow onion, thinly sliced

2 cups cauliflower florets

¼ cup sliced green onions, white and green parts

1. Preheat the oven to 425°F. Lightly grease a rimmed baking sheet with sesame or olive oil, and set aside.

2. In a small bowl, combine the tahini, miso paste, coconut aminos, vinegar, and sweetener.

3. Pour the mixture into a zip-top bag and add the tempeh. Marinate for at least 20 minutes, or overnight.

4. In a large bowl, add the Brussels sprouts, yellow onion, cauliflower florets, and green onion. Add the tempeh and marinade to the vegetables, and toss to combine.

5. Transfer the tempeh to the baking sheet, and bake for 10 to 15 minutes.

6. Turn the vegetables over, and bake an additional 15 minutes, until the tempeh is golden brown, and all the vegetables are tender.

7. Tranfser to individual bowls and serve.

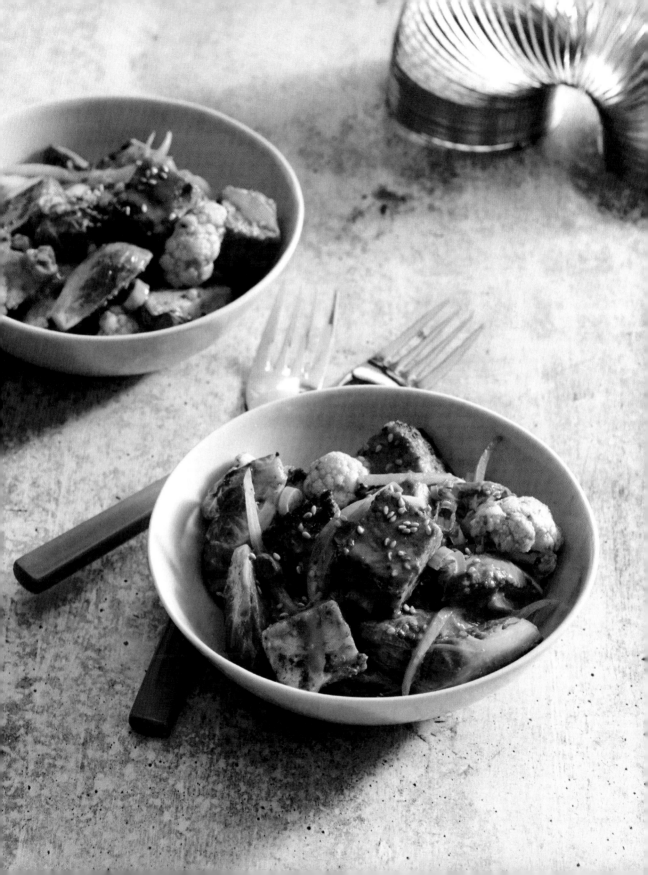

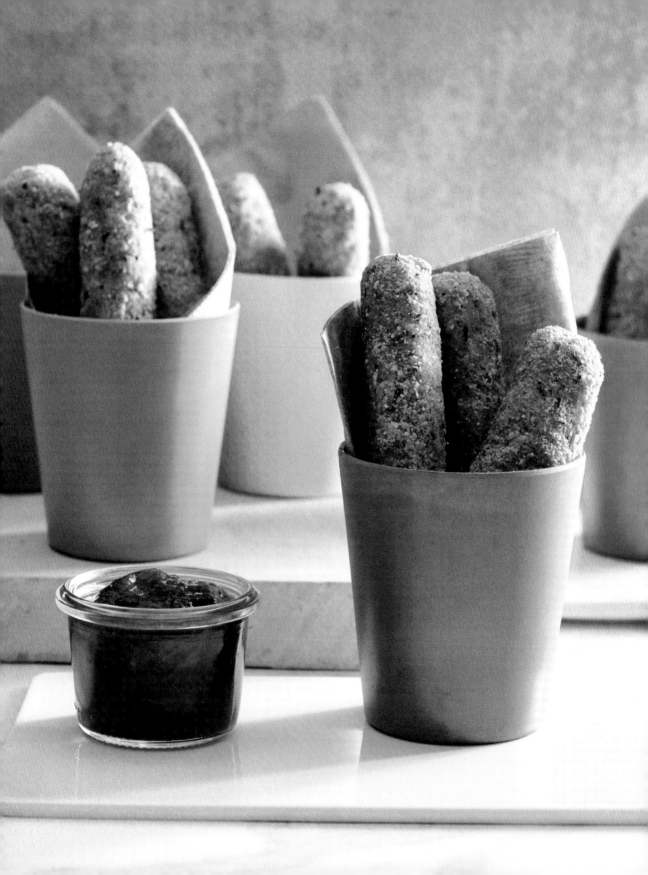

Hearts of Palm "Fish" Sticks

Here is a healthy, delicious take on the popular from-the-box food kids love, fish sticks. Instead of fish, I like to use gut-boosting hearts of palm and mix it up with flavorful parmesan, herbs, and spices. These come together fast—and they'll disappear from your dinner table even faster!

SERVES 4-6

100% olive oil cooking spray (to cook in oven)

2 14-ounce cans hearts of palm, well drained

½ cup shredded Parmigiano-Reggiano or nutritional yeast

¼ cup fresh Italian parsley

½ cup ground flaxseed

1 tablespoon Old Bay Seasoning

½ teaspoon paprika

½ teaspoon oregano

¼ teaspoon freshly ground black pepper

1 sushi-size sheet of seaweed (nori)

½ cup tapioca starch

1 cup almond flour

2 large omega-3 eggs

Sea salt, to serve

Tangy Ranch Dressing/Dip (page 219)

Lectin-Light Ketchup (page 220)

1. Line a rimmed baking sheet with parchment, and set aside.

2. In the bowl of a food processor fitted with an S-blade, add the hearts of palm, Parmigiano-Reggiano, parsley, flaxseed, Old Bay, paprika, oregano, black pepper, and nori and pulse until well combined. Let rest for 5 to 10 minutes to let the flaxseeds thicken the mixture.

3. Check to see if you can mold the mixture into "sticks" with your hands—if yes, skip to Step 5.

4. If the mixture is too thin to mold into sticks, add the tapioca starch, 1 tablespoon at a time. If too thick, add water, a tablespoon at a time, and keep blending until "moldable."

5. Shape the hearts of palm mixture into "sticks" and place on the prepared baking sheet. (It's okay if you can't pick up the sticks at this point, just aim for approximately the right shape and size.)

6. Freeze the sticks for 15 to 30 minutes until they are easy to handle.

7. Meanwhile, in a small bowl, whisk together the remaining tapioca starch and almond flour.

8. In a separate bowl, whisk together the eggs.

9. Dip each frozen "fish" stick in the egg mixture, then in the flour mixture, coating evenly, and set aside. If they do not feel as firm as you'd like, freeze them again.

10. Cook the sticks using one of the two methods below.

TO COOK IN THE OVEN:

1. Spray a rimmed baking sheet with oil, and place in a cold oven. Preheat the oven (and baking sheet) to 425°F.

2. When the baking sheet is hot, spray with an additional coating of oil. Transfer the "fish" sticks to the baking sheet, spreading in a single layer, and spray the tops with olive oil.

3. Bake for 8 to 10 minutes, then flip, and bake for another 4 to 5 minutes, until heated through. Sprinkle with the salt after cooking.

4. Serve with the ranch dressing. ketchup, and a great big green salad.

TO COOK IN AN AIR FRYER:

1. Preheat the air fryer to 380°F.

2. Spray the fryer basket with olive oil, and arrange the "fish" sticks in a single layer in the basket—you may need to cook in batches.

3. Cook for 5 to 6 minutes, then flip the "fish" sticks and cook for an additional 5 to 6 minutes. Sprinkle with the salt after cooking.

4. Serve with the ranch dressing, ketchup, and a great big green salad.

chapter seven

Instantly Delicious

Not-Too-Spicy Tikka Masala

Chicken Tikka Masala is one of the most popular dishes in Indian restaurants, and for good reason: it is absolutely delicious. When you're scanning the ingredients list here and see tomato paste and puree, don't be alarmed—pressure cooking takes care of the lectins. If you're planning to cook on the stovetop, omit the tomato paste and puree and instead add an additional cup of coconut milk or yogurt for a super rich and creamy curry.

SERVES 4

1 pound boneless, skinless pastured chicken thighs or jackfruit

1 ½ teaspoons kosher salt, divided

1 tablespoon grass-fed butter or olive oil

1 small yellow onion, minced

4 cloves garlic, minced

1 tablespoon fresh minced ginger

1 ½ tablespoons garam masala

1 teaspoon cayenne pepper (optional, for heat)

2 teaspoons cumin

1 tablespoon turmeric

1 tablespoon tomato paste*

1 cup plain tomato puree*

2 13.6 oz cans full-fat coconut milk

1 cup cauliflower florets

1 cup coconut or goat's milk yogurt

Juice of 1 lemon

Cauliflower rice or Perfect Basmati Rice (page 231), for serving

1. Cut the chicken into bite-sized chunks, and season with ½ teaspoon kosher salt. Set aside.

2. Add butter or oil to the Instant Pot, set to sauté, and heat the oil. Add onion, garlic, ginger, garam masala, cayenne, cumin, and turmeric.

3. Cook, stirring frequently, until onion is soft and mixture is very fragrant.

4. Add tomato paste, and cook an additional minute, stirring until well-combined.

5. Add chicken, and saute until just browned, about 4 to 5 minutes.

6. Add tomato puree, then open the cans of coconut milk. Carefully spoon out the thick cream, and set it aside.

7. Add ¾ cup of the thinner, watery "milk" from the coconut milk to the Instant Pot, as well as the remaining salt.

8. Cover, and cook on high pressure for 10 minutes, then then release pressure with a quick release.

9. Uncover, and stir in the coconut cream set aside earlier, and cauliflower florets, then turn the Instant Pot to sauté. Bring to a simmer, and cook until thickened, about 15 minutes.

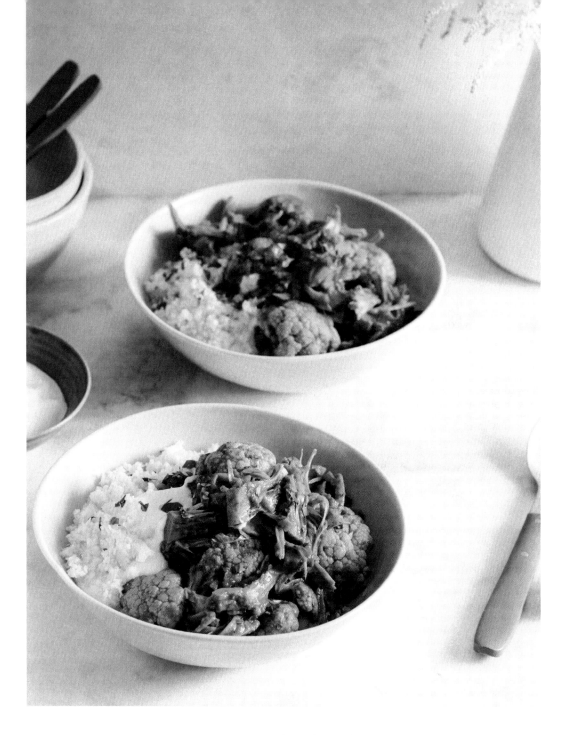

10. Remove from heat, then stir in the yogurt and lemon juice before serving over cauliflower rice or Perfect Basmati Rice.

"Spaghetti" and Meatballs

The classic, Italian-inspired version of spaghetti and meatballs is high in lectins, from the tomato sauce to the wheat flour pasta to the breadcrumbs in the meatballs. Luckily, there are simple swaps that can make this beloved dish as good for you as it is tasty. You can use a gluten-free pasta here (I like Cappello's) or spiralized sweet potato noodles. If you are avoiding meat, feel free to substitute additional mushrooms or ground tempeh for the "meatballs."

SERVES 4

1 pound mushrooms

2 shallots or ½ red onion

½ cup grated Parmigiano-Reggiano

2 cloves garlic

½ pound ground grass-fed beef, lamb, or turkey

2 large omega-3 eggs or flaxseed eggs*

6 tablespoons cassava flour

4 tablespoons flaxseed meal

1 teaspoon sea salt

½ teaspoon garlic powder

½ teaspoon oregano

½ teaspoon dried basil

½ teaspoon paprika

¼ cup olive oil

3 cups Dr. G's Tomato Sauce (page 221)

2 cups Cappello's pasta cooked according to package instructions, or spiralized cooked spiralized sweet potatoes**

1. To make the meatballs, in the bowl of a food processor fitted with an S-blade, pulse together the mushrooms, shallots or onion, Parmigiano-Reggiano, and garlic until a paste is formed.

2. Transfer the paste to a bowl, and fold in the meat, eggs, cassava flour, flaxseed meal, salt, garlic powder, oregano, basil, and paprika.

3. Using your hands or a spring-loaded ice cream scoop, shape the mixture into bite-size balls. If the mixture is too loose, add additional cassava flour, a spoonful at a time, until cohesive.

4. Once the meatballs are shaped, freeze them for 10 minutes—this helps them really keep their shape.

5. Add oil to the Instant Pot, set to sauté, and heat the oil. Add the meatballs to the pot in a single layer. You may have to work in batches.

6. Brown the meatballs on all sides, then add the tomato sauce.

7. Lock the lid, and cook on high pressure for 7 minutes. Release the pressure with a quick release.

8. Serve over the cooked pasta or sweet potato "noodles."

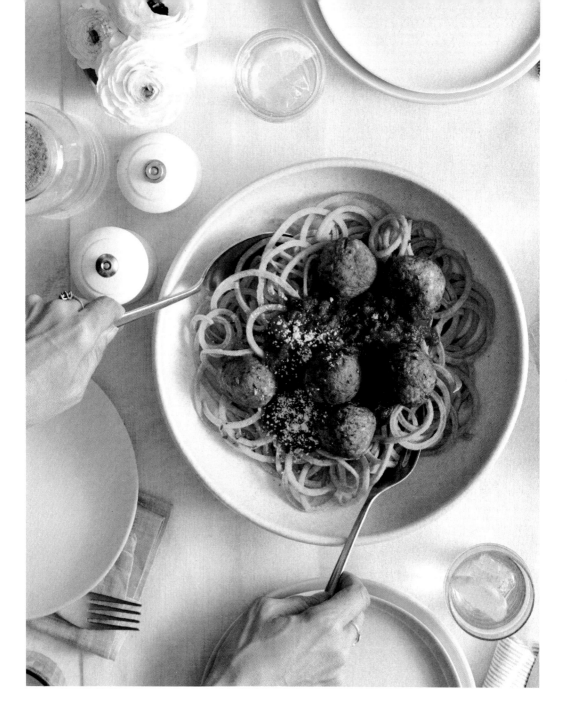

*To make a flaxseed egg, combine 1 tablespoon of ground flaxseed with 3 tablespoons water, and let sit at least 10 minutes before using.

**Pour 2 Tbsp of olive oil into a large skillet and heat over medium high heat. When oil is hot, add the spiralized sweet potatos and toss to coat with the oil. Cook, tossing every few seconds, for 5-10 minutes (5 for a more "al dente" noodle, 10 for a softer one.

Sweet Potato Noodle Lasagna

Here is a delicious lasagna, but instead of regular pasta, thin slices of sweet potato stand in for noodles. The best part is that the whole thing cooks in your Instant Pot in just 30 minutes and comes out moist, delicate, and so delicious! For a crispy top, finish the lasagna in the oven under the broiler.

SERVES 8

100% olive oil cooking spray

¼ cup extra-virgin olive oil

1 yellow onion, diced

1 bag Quorn crumbles or 12 ounces ground grass-fed beef

4 cloves garlic, minced

1 teaspoon sea salt

½ teaspoon freshly ground black pepper

2 cups Dr. G's Tomato Sauce (page 221)

2 cups goat's or sheep's milk ricotta or 3 cups coconut yogurt

½ teaspoon dried oregano

Zest and juice of 1 lemon

½ cup basil pesto

2 large omega-3 or free-range eggs or 2 VeganEggs

½ cup grated Parmigiano-Reggiano

1 large sweet potato, very thinly sliced (this will be your noodles)

1. Spray a heatproof ceramic or springform dish that fits into your Instant Pot with oil, and set aside.

2. And the oil to your Instant Pot, set to sauté, and heat the oil.

3. Add the onion and Quorn crumbles, and cook, stirring occasionally, until the onion is translucent, about 5 minutes.

4. Then add the garlic, salt, and pepper, and continue to cook, until the garlic is fragrant.

5. Add the tomato sauce and simmer until the sauce is thickened, about 10 minutes, then set aside. (Rinse your Instant Pot if necessary.)

6. In a large bowl, mix together the ricotta, oregano, lemon zest and juice, basil pesto, eggs, and two thirds of the Parmigiano-Reggiano, and set aside.

7. To assemble your lasagna in the prepared container, spoon ½ cup tomato sauce into the base of your baking dish, and layer on one layer of the thinly-sliced sweet potato "noodles."

8. Top with ½ cup ricotta mixture.

9. Repeat steps 7 and 8, until the pan is full (3 to 4 layers).

10. Sprinkle the top of the lasagna with the remaining Parmigiano-Reggiano.

11. Pour 1½ cups water into your Instant Pot, and add the steaming shelf.

12. Place the prepared lasagna on top of the shelf, and set for "manual cook" for 30 minutes. Let the pressure release manually.

13. Serve as is, or briefly broil in the oven if you prefer a crispy crust.

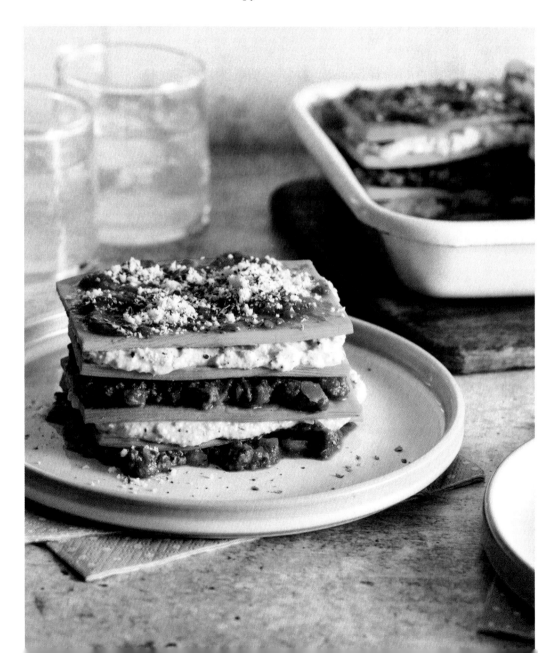

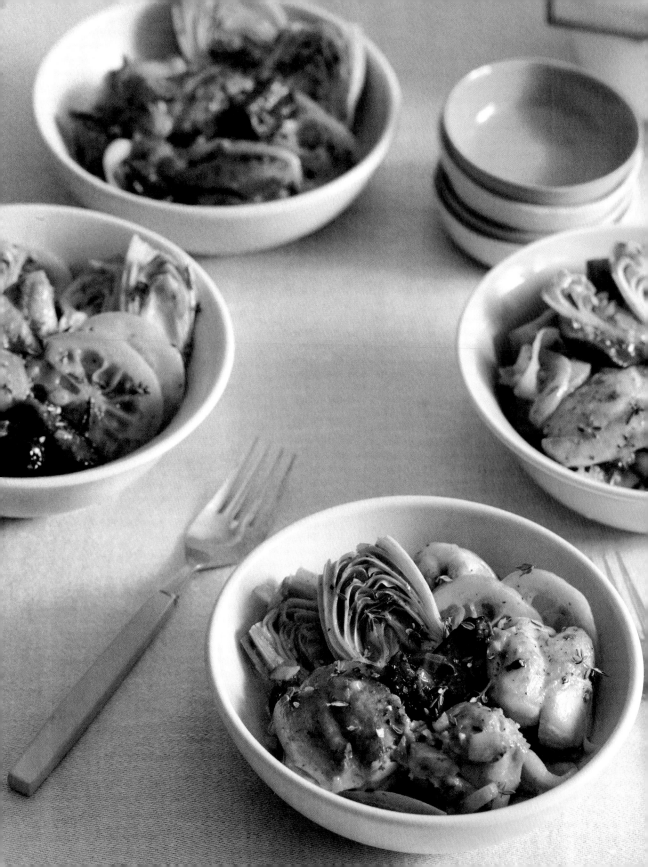

Braised Chicken with Artichokes

In this crowd-pleasing dish, Mediterranean flavors meld together in the Instant Pot to deliver a stunningly fragrant and tasty dinner that tastes like it took hours to prepare. If you can't find fresh artichokes, frozen ones will do in a pinch, and will save prep time, but avoid using canned artichokes, which will become mushy.

SERVES 4

1½ teaspoons salt, divided

½ teaspoon freshly ground black pepper

½ teaspoon smoked paprika

1 pound pasture-raised boneless, skinless chicken thigh meat, cut into bite-size chunks

¼ cup extra-virgin olive oil

1 large onion, minced

4 cloves garlic, minced

1 tablespoon fresh thyme

1 tablespoon fresh rosemary

½ cup dried figs, diced

4 cups quartered artichoke hearts (frozen, or canned and rinsed)

1 lemon, thinly sliced

2 cups chicken broth

3 tablespoons tapioca starch (optional)

¼ cup water (optional)

1. Set your Instant Pot to sauté.

2. While the pot is heating, whisk together ½ teaspoon of the salt, the black pepper, and the paprika. Season the chicken liberally with the mixture.

3. Heat the oil in the Instant Pot and add the onion, garlic, thyme, rosemary, and the remaining salt. Cook, stirring frequently, until the onion is tender.

4. Add the chicken, and sear until golden brown on all sides.

5. Then add the figs, artichoke hearts, lemon, and broth to your Instant Pot.

6. Lock the lid into place, and cook on high pressure for 7 minutes. Release pressure with a quick release and serve the chicken and artichokes, spooning the sauce over top.

7. If you would prefer a thicker sauce, switch the pot back to sauté. In a small bowl, whisk together the tapioca starch and water, then add to the pot.

8. Cook, stirring frequently, until the sauce reaches desired consistency. Serve immediately.

Portobello "Pot Roast"

The Plant Paradox spin on pot roast uses portobello mushrooms, cauliflower, and sweet potatoes in place of beef. I daresay this is even more comforting and satisfying than the original version, perfect for colder nights when you just want something warm and nourishing.

SERVES 4 TO 6

¼ cup extra-virgin olive oil, divided

6 large portobello mushrooms, cut into chunks

2 cups cauliflower florets

1 large onion, minced

2 large sweet potatoes, diced

3 cloves garlic, minced

1 teaspoon sea salt, plus more to taste

½ teaspoon freshly ground black pepper

¼ teaspoon sweet paprika

1½ cups good-quality white wine

¼ cup coconut aminos

2 cups vegetable or mushroom broth

2 sprigs fresh thyme

1 large sprig fresh rosemary

4 tablespoons tapioca starch or arrowroot powder

4 tablespoons cold water

1. Set your Instant Pot to sauté, and add half of the oil. Add the mushrooms and cauliflower, and cook, stirring occasionally, until golden brown. Transfer to a plate.

2. Add the remaining oil to the pot, and sauté the onion until golden brown. Add the sweet potatoes, and continue to cook, until just starting to brown at the edges.

3. Next add the garlic, salt, black pepper, and paprika, and sauté for an additional minute, until the garlic is fragrant.

4. Then add the wine, coconut aminos, broth, thyme, and rosemary, and stir to combine, scraping the bottom of the pot to loosen any flavorful bits.

5. Place the lid on the Instant Pot, seal, and cook on manual (pressure cook) for 10 minutes. Let the pressure release naturally.

6. Meanwhile, in a small bowl, whisk together the tapioca starch and water until smooth and milky looking.

7. Remove the herb sprigs from the Instant Pot, and turn it back to sauté.

8. Pour in the starch mixture and the mushroom and cauliflower mixture, and whisk to incorporate. When the sauce is thickened and the mushroom/cauliflower mixture is hot, serve.

Lamb (or Mushroom) Curry

Don't let the long list of ingredients scare you off; this curry is easy to make and delivers so much flavor, you might want to cook a double batch. As with most stews, this dish tastes even better the next day, so consider making it a day before you plan on serving it, maybe on a Sunday afternoon for a Monday or Tuesday dinner. Garam masala is an Indian blend of spices, available at grocery stores or online. For a vegetarian curry, use 1½ pounds of chopped portobello mushrooms instead of the lamb.

SERVES 4

¼ cup extra-virgin olive oil

1 pound boneless lamb shoulder or leg, trimmed and cubed

2 large onions, minced

4 cloves garlic, minced

1 tablespoon fresh minced ginger

1 teaspoon sea salt

1½ tablespoons garam masala

1 tablespoon turmeric

1 teaspoon cumin

½ teaspoon ground coriander

½ teaspoon freshly ground black pepper

½ teaspoon cinnamon

¼ teaspoon ground cardamom

¼ teaspoon cayenne pepper

¼ cup almond butter

1 can full-fat coconut milk

1 cup mushroom broth

3 cups cauliflower florets

Juice of 1 small lemon

4 cups fresh baby spinach, rinsed and dried

1. Set your Instant Pot to sauté, and heat the oil.

2. When hot, add the lamb and brown on all sides, then transfer to a plate.

3. Add the onions and sauté until translucent and tender, then add the garlic, ginger, salt, and the spices.

4. Cook until very fragrant, then add the almond butter, and stir until combined.

5. Place the lamb back into the pot, along with the coconut milk and broth.

6. Seal the pot, and cook on high pressure for 20 minutes (3 minutes for mushrooms, if using).

7. Allow the pressure to release naturally for 10 minutes, then quick release the pressure the rest of the way.

8. Remove the lid, add the cauliflower and lemon juice, and simmer for about 15 minutes, until the cauliflower is tender.

9. Add the spinach and stir until it is just wilted, then serve.

Perfect Roast Chicken and Vegetables

Roast chicken is delicious, but hard to accomplish on a weeknight—it takes well over an hour to get your chicken from oven to table. That's hard to manage when you have a hungry family to feed! Enter the Instant Pot, which cooks your chicken in mere minutes, thus making a beautiful roast chicken a reality for your weeknight dinners. If you prefer crispy skin, finish the chicken under the broiler for a few minutes. For a vegetarian option, try roasting a whole head of cauliflower this way.

SERVES 4 TO 6

1 whole, skin-on pasture-raised chicken, 2.5 to 3 lbs*

1 lemon, quartered

2 bay leaves

1 sprig rosemary

1 teaspoon sea salt, divided

¼ cup extra-virgin olive oil, divided

1 large onion, sliced

4 ribs celery, sliced

2 cups sliced mushrooms

½ teaspoon freshly ground black pepper

1 tablespoon fresh thyme

1 tablespoon fresh sage

1 cup white wine or chicken broth

1. To prepare the chicken, stuff the cavity with the lemon, bay leaves, and rosemary, and tie with butchers' twine, making sure it will fit in your Instant Pot.

2. Season with ½ teaspoon of the salt.

3. Set your Instant Pot to sauté, and heat half of the oil. Sear the chicken, breast side down, until golden brown, then carefully sear the legs, using tongs to position the chicken.

4. Remove the chicken from the Instant Pot and add the remaining oil.

5. Add the onion, celery, and mushrooms, along with the remaining salt, the pepper, thyme, and sage, and briefly sauté until the onion is translucent.

6. Place the chicken breast side up on top of the vegetables, add wine or broth, and cook on manual (pressure cook) for 8 minutes per pound of chicken.

7. Let the pressure release naturally, then remove the chicken and vegetables from the Instant Pot.

8. Serve immediately, or place the chicken under the broiler for a few minutes to crisp up the skin before serving with the vegetables.

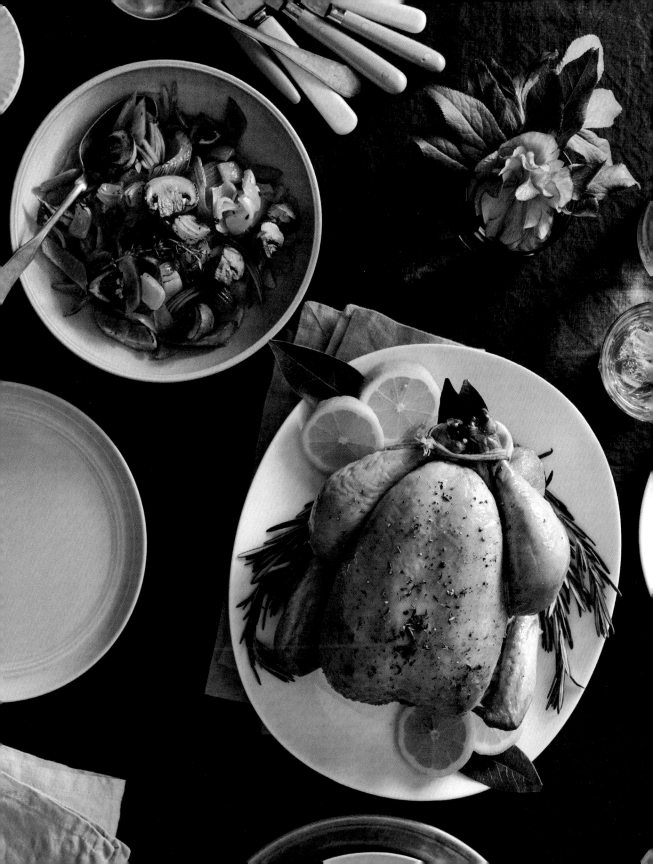

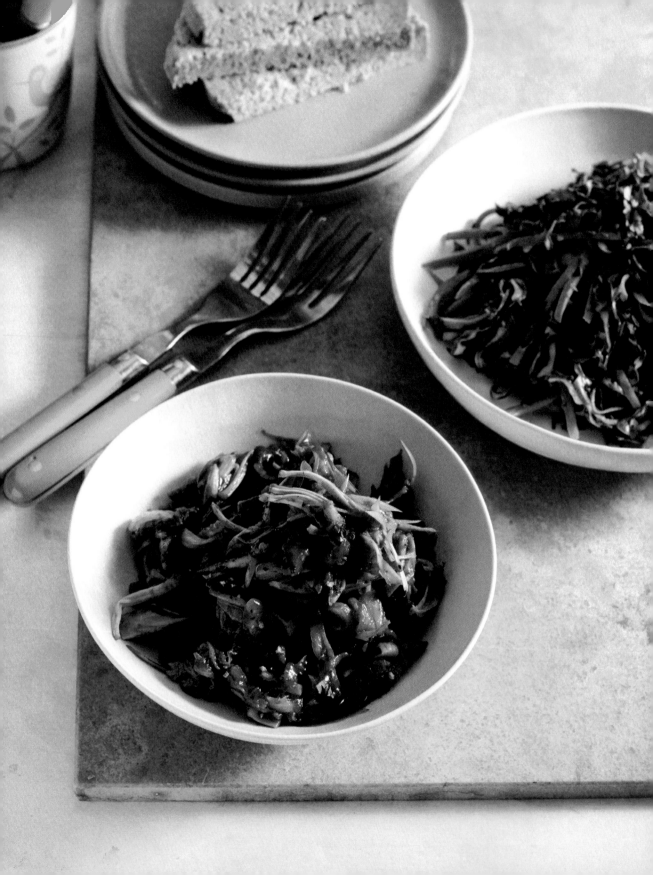

BBQ Pulled Pork

Look for pasture-raised pork shoulder (also known as Boston butt) to make this easy dish that is perfect for potlucks and parties. Serve the meat with a simple slaw and my Cauliflower "Mac" and Cheese (page 115) to recreate a classic barbecue plate that tastes great, but is a lot better for you. For a vegetarian option, you can use jackfruit that has been canned in brine, or frozen. I would avoid fresh jackfruit, as it requires extensive preparation.

SERVES 4 TO 6

1½ pounds pork shoulder or jackfruit (core removed)

1 teaspoon sea salt

1 teaspoon smoked paprika

1 teaspoon garlic powder

½ teaspoon cumin

¼ teaspoon cinnamon

2 large onions, thinly sliced

3 cups Almost Classic BBQ Sauce (page 215)

1. Cut the pork shoulder in half, so that it easily fits into your Instant Pot.

2. In a small bowl, combine the salt, paprika, garlic powder, cumin, and cinnamon.

3. Rub the pork shoulder with the seasoning mix, and transfer to your Instant Pot, along with the onions and barbecue sauce.

4. Cook for 45 minutes for pork (6 minutes for jackfruit).

5. Serve with sides of your choice, and enjoy.

Thai Coconut Chicken

Thai curries are delightfully flavorful, though they usually require a lot of time to slowly simmer on the stove. Using a pressure cooker, my coconut chicken comes together in no time. Note that red curry paste and fish sauce are available at most supermarkets these days, as well as online. When buying canned coconut milk, always look for varieties that contain only coconut and water, without any additives. For vegetarian option, swap tempeh for the chicken.

SERVES 4 TO 6

¼ cup sesame or avocado oil

1 pound pasture-raised skinless chicken, cut into bite-size pieces

1 large onion, thinly sliced

5 cloves garlic, sliced

2 tablespoons minced ginger

2 tablespoons Thai red curry paste

1 can full-fat coconut milk

3 tablespoons fish sauce or 6 tablespoons coconut aminos

1 tablespoon monk fruit sweetener or local honey

2 cups very small cauliflower florets

2 cups very small broccoli florets

2 cups sliced bok choy or cabbage

1 tablespoon lime juice

½ cup Thai basil leaves

½ cup cilantro leaves

1. Set your Instant Pot to sauté, and heat the oil.

2. Add the chicken, onion, garlic, and ginger, and sauté until the chicken is browned and the onion is very tender, about 5 to 7 minutes.

3. Next add the curry paste and cook an additional minute.

4. Then add the coconut milk, fish sauce, and sweetener to the pot, and stir to combine.

5. Seal the pot, and cook on high pressure—8 minutes for white meat, 10 minutes for dark meat.

6. Release the pressure with a quick release, and add the cauliflower, broccoli, and bok choy.

7. Switch the pot to sauté and simmer for 5 to 7 minutes, until the vegetables are tender.

8. Add the lime juice, basil leaves, and cilantro right before serving.

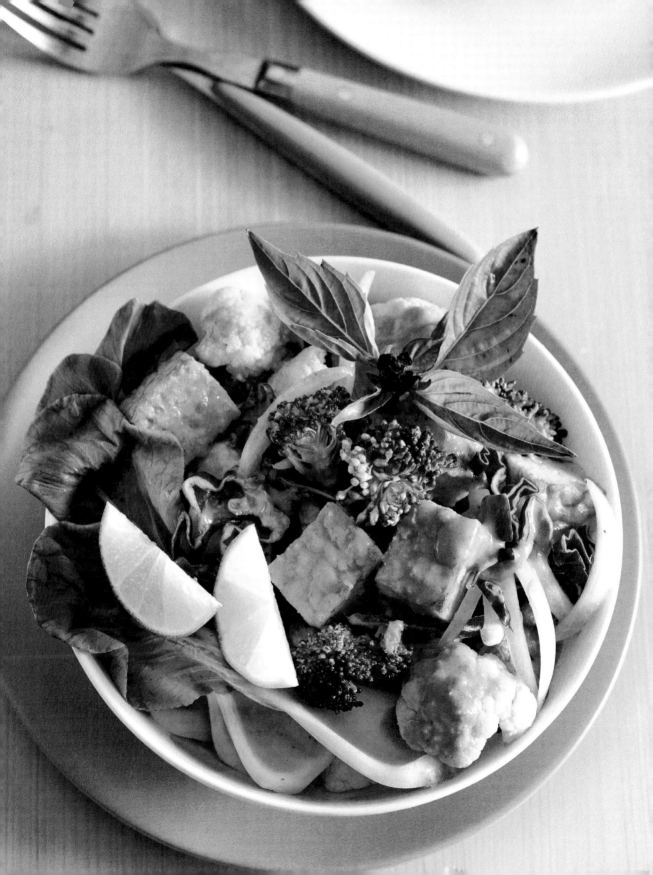

chapter eight

Satisfying Soups

Broccoli Cheddar Soup

My variation on this much-beloved classic uses goat's milk cheddar place of cow's milk cheese, but keeps intact all of the creamy indulgence of the original. To make a vegan soup, omit the cheddar and use about a cup of nutritional yeast (you'll need to add a little extra salt as well), and be sure to choose vegetable stock. Serve this soup with a simple green salad on a chilly day, and prepare to feel thoroughly cozy.

SERVES 4

¼ cup extra-virgin olive oil

3 cups broccoli florets

1 yellow onion, minced

2 ribs celery, diced

3 cloves garlic, minced

1 teaspoon sea salt

1 teaspoon black pepper

1 teaspoon powdered mustard

1 can coconut cream or full-fat coconut milk

4 cups chicken or vegetable broth

1 cup shredded goat's milk Cheddar*

Coconut aminos to taste

Chopped green onions, for serving

1. Set your Instant Pot to sauté, and heat the oil.

2. Add the broccoli, onion, celery, garlic, salt, pepper, and powdered mustard, and cook, stirring frequently, until the onion is translucent.

3. Then add the coconut cream and broth, and seal the pot. Cook on high pressure for 8 minutes, then carefully release the pressure using a quick release—there will be a lot of steam.

4. Switch the Instant Pot back to sauté, and add the Cheddar, a small handful at a time, stirring until it melts.

5. Taste, and add the coconut aminos as needed. Serve garnished with the green onions.

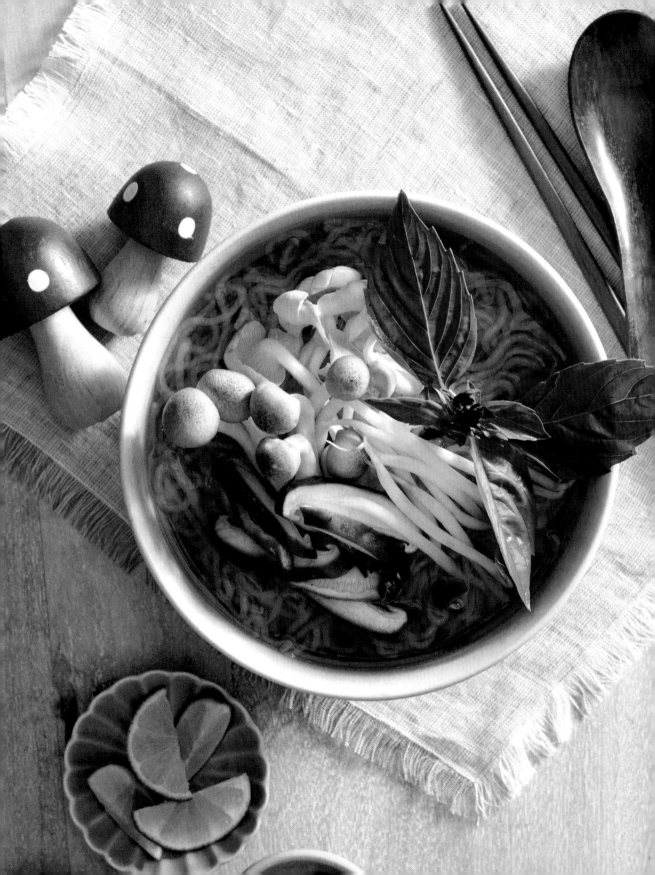

Miracle Noodle Pho

This is the perfect soup to eat when you're under the weather or when you just want a bit of comfort. Fragrant from spices such as star anise and cloves, and imbued with garlic and ginger, this broth is good enough to sip on its own, but is made even better by the addition of miracle noodles.

SERVES 4 TO 6

2 cups peeled, cubed daikon radishes

2 onions, quartered

½ green cabbage, cut into chunks

6 cloves garlic

1 4-inch chunk of ginger, cut in half lengthwise

1 tablespoon avocado oil

3 cups chopped mushrooms (oyster, cremini, shiitake, or portobello are great)

8 cups mushroom stock

4 to 5 pieces star anise

1 tablespoon whole coriander seeds

3 pods cardamom

1 3- to 4-inch cinnamon stick

1 teaspoon whole cloves

2 packs miracle noodles, rinsed and boiled to get rid of smell

1 cup cilantro, for serving

1 cup basil, for serving

Juice of 2 limes, for serving

Fish sauce or coconut aminos to taste

1. In a large skillet, over high heat, char your radishes, onions, cabbage, garlic, and ginger until basically blackened.

2. While charring, set your Instant Pot to sauté, and heat the oil. Add the mushrooms and sauté until tender.

3. Transfer the charred mixture to the Instant Pot with the mushrooms, and gradually fill with the stock, making sure the liquid level is under the "max fill" line.

4. Add the star anise, coriander seeds, cardamom, cinnamon stick, and whole cloves. (The spices can be wrapped in a piece of cheesecloth for easy removal.)

5. Seal the pot, and pressure cook for 15 minutes. Release pressure naturally (there will be a lot of steam).

6. With a slotted spoon, strain out the charred ingredients and spices, leaving just the stock and mushrooms.

7. Add the miracle noodles, and let simmer for 10 minutes.

8. Serve garnished with the cilantro, basil, and lime juice. Season with the fish sauce or coconut aminos.

Creamy Leek and Potato Soup

Leek and potato soup is a quintessential winter meal, but it's also delicious served chilled in warmer months. Using cauliflower in place of potatoes keeps the soup creamy while lessening its lectin content, and leeks are a probiotic-rich food our gut buddies love to feast on—plus they add terrific flavor. Just be sure to wash your leeks well before using, getting in between the leaves where grit is often trapped.

SERVES 6 TO 8

¼ cup extra-virgin olive oil

3 leeks, rinsed of grit and thinly chopped

1 celery root, diced

2 parsnips, peeled and diced

1 cup diced cauliflower

1 russet potato, peeled and diced

1½ teaspoons sea salt

1 teaspoon freshly ground white pepper

1 bay leaf

3 sprigs thyme, more for garnish

6 to 8 cups chicken or vegetable broth, divided

1. Set your Instant Pot to sauté, and heat the oil.

2. Add the leeks, celery root, parsnips, and cauliflower and cook until the leeks begin to wilt, about 5 minutes.

3. Then add the potato, salt, pepper, bay leaf, thyme, and 6 cups broth, and cook on high pressure for 12 minutes, then release pressure with a manual release.

4. Remove bay leaf and thyme sprigs.

5. Using an immersion blender (or transfer to a high-speed blender), blend the soup until smooth. Add more broth as needed to reach your desired consistency.

6. Taste, and add salt as needed before serving.

Green Chili with Chicken

Green chili, or *chili verde*, gets its name from the color of the chili peppers used in the dish, but I've included plenty of other "greens" in here as well, including spinach, cilantro, and avocado. Unlike traditional chilis, green chili typically doesn't contain beans, so making it lectin-free is relatively easy. When we cook this at home we sometimes load it up with extra vegetables and add just a little bit of chicken for protein. You can serve it on its own or over cauliflower rice.

SERVES 4 TO 6

4 cups cauliflower florets

2 cups baby spinach

1 cup cilantro, stems and leaves separated

6½ cups chicken or vegetable broth

3 tablespoon extra-virgin olive oil

1 large celery root (celeriac), peeled

2 large onions, diced

3 pasilla or Anaheim chilis, peeled, seeded, and diced

1½ teaspoons sea salt

2 teaspoons cumin

2 teaspoons garlic powder

½ teaspoon freshly ground black pepper

1½ pounds boneless, skinless chicken thighs or jackfruit

Zest and juice of 2 limes

½ cup sugar-free salsa verde

1 diced avocado, for serving

1. In your Instant Pot, add the cauliflower, spinach, cilantro stems, and 1½ cups chicken broth.

2. Seal the pot, and cook for 2 minutes on high pressure. Release the pressure immediately.

3. Transfer the mixture to a blender, blend until smooth, and set aside.

4. In the Instant Pot, add the oil, celery root, onions, chilis, salt, cumin, garlic powder, and black pepper. Cook on sauté for about 5 minutes, until the onions are tender.

5. Add the chicken thighs, the remaining broth, lime zest, and salsa verde.

6. Seal the pot, and cook on high pressure for 13 minutes. Release the pressure with a quick release, being careful of the steam. Remove the chicken, and shred with two forks.

7. Add the chicken back to the pot, along with the blended cauliflower mixture, lime juice, and cilantro leaves.

8. Taste, and add salt if needed. Serve topped with the diced avocado.

Bean and Mushroom Chili

Your eyes aren't deceiving you: This is a traditional chili of beans, tomatoes, and peppers! Pressure-cooking these ingredients in the Instant Pot takes care of the lectins and makes them safe to consume. I love the heft and umami flavor the mushrooms add, and the earthy sweetness imparted by flavonoid-rich cocoa powder creates another layer of rich, traditional "chili" flavor.

SERVES 6

¼ cup olive oil

1 large onion, chopped

5 cloves garlic, minced

3 ribs celery, minced

3 cups diced mushrooms

1 to 2 poblano peppers, peeled, seeded, and chopped

6 large tomatoes, peeled, seeded, and minced*

Zest of 1 orange

3 tablespoons chili powder

2 tablespoons natural cocoa powder

1 tablespoon ground cumin

1 teaspoon freshly ground black pepper

½ teaspoon ground cinnamon

¼ teaspoon ground cloves

1 teaspoon sea salt

1½ cups dried pinto beans

1½ cups dried black beans

6 cups water or vegetable broth

1 diced avocado, to serve

1 cup chopped cilantro, to serve (optional)

Or 1 28-ounce can Italian diced tomatoes (peeled and seeded).

1. Set your Instant Pot to sauté, and heat the oil.

2. Sauté the onion, garlic, celery, mushrooms, and peppers until very fragrant, about 5 to 8 minutes.

3. Add the tomatoes, orange zest, chili powder, cocoa powder, cumin, black pepper, cinnamon, cloves, and salt, and sauté an additional 1 to 2 minutes.

4. Then add the pinto and black beans and water or broth, seal the pot, and cook for 20 minutes at pressure.

5. Let the pressure release naturally, then stir. Taste, and add salt as needed.

6. To serve, garnish with the avocado and cilantro, if using.

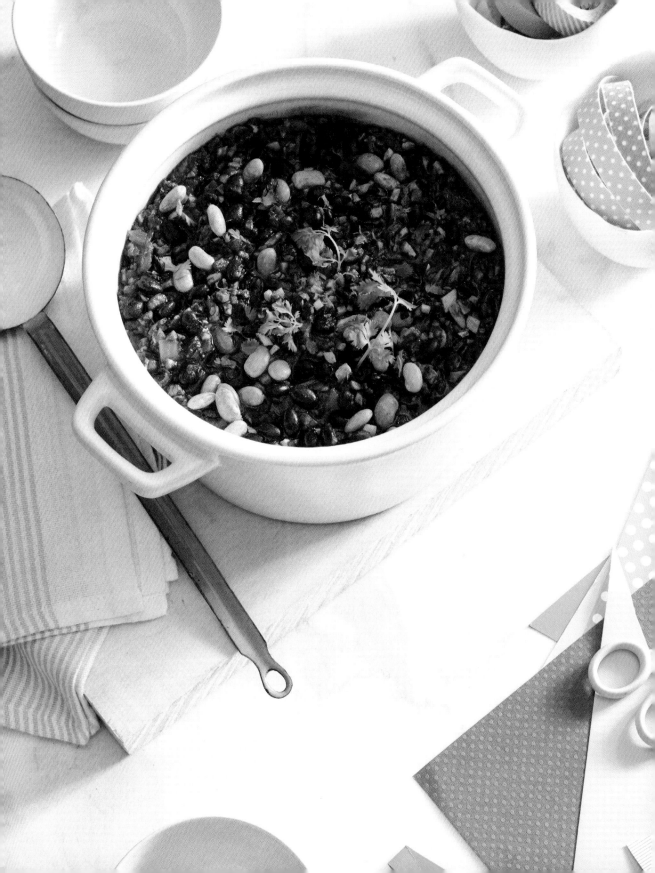

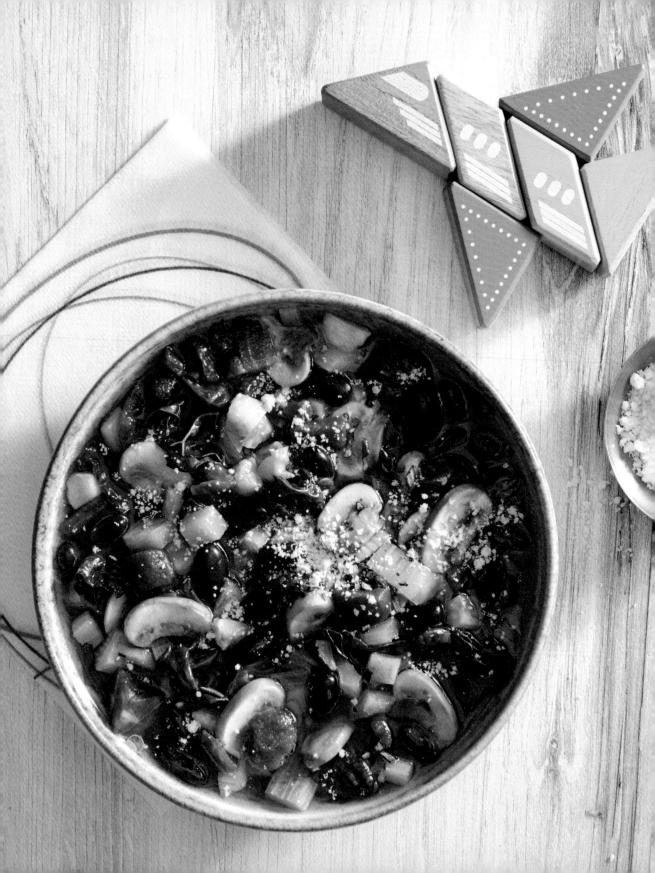

Minestrone Soup

This soup is comfort in a bowl. Using a pressure cooker is key to removing the lectins from the tomatoes and beans, so be sure to cook this one as directed. I love the flavor of fennel in this soup—combined with the basil and oregano, it really feels like an authentic Italian dish. Make a big batch and freeze in jars for easy, single-serving meals.

SERVES 6-8

¼ cup extra-virgin olive oil

1 onion, diced

3 stalks celery, diced

1 pound fennel, diced

1½ teaspoons sea salt

3 cloves garlic, minced

2 cups minced mushrooms

1½ teaspoons dried basil

1 teaspoon dried oregano

2 tablespoons fresh minced rosemary

6 cups chicken or vegetable broth

1 28-ounce can diced Italian tomatoes

1 cup dried kidney beans, soaked in 2 to 3 changes of water

1 large Parmigiano-Reggiano rind

1 bay leaf

1 bunch kale, stems removed and leaves chopped

1 tablespoon red wine vinegar or lemon juice

1. Set your Instant Pot to sauté, and heat the oil. Add the onion, celery, fennel, and 1 teaspoon salt, and cook, stirring frequently, until tender.

2. Add the garlic and mushrooms, and cook an additional couple of minutes, until the garlic is incredibly fragrant.

3. Then add the basil, oregano, rosemary, and the remaining sea salt and sauté until very fragrant.

4. Add the broth, tomatoes, kidney beans, Parmigiano-Reggiano rind, and bay leaf.

5. Seal the pot and cook at high pressure for 20 minutes.

6. Release pressure with a quick release, being aware of the steam.

7. Add the kale, and stir until wilted, about 5 minutes.

8. Then add the vinegar or lemon juice, taste, and season with additional salt, as needed. Ladle into bowls and serve.

Split Pea and Vegetable Soup

This vegetable-packed split pea soup is as delicious and flavorful as any you've had before—and a whole lot healthier. You'll need to soak the split peas overnight, ideally changing the water at least once before using. I like to add a bit of prosciutto to my soup to get that rich, salty flavor, but if you're a vegetarian or vegan, feel free to omit it.

SERVES 6

1 cup water or chicken broth

2 cups cauliflower florets

2 cups baby spinach

3 tablespoons extra-virgin olive oil

1 large onion, minced

3 stalks celery, minced

4 cloves garlic, chopped

2 bay leaves, chopped

¼ teaspoon freshly ground black pepper

1 teaspoon smoked paprika

6 to 8 cups water, chicken broth, or vegetable broth

½ pound dried split peas, soaked in 1 to 2 changes of water

½ teaspoon salt

½ cup sliced prosciutto (optional)

1. In your Instant Pot, add the water or broth, cauliflower, and spinach. Seal the pot, and cook at high pressure for 5 minutes.

2. Release pressure manually, then transfer the mixture to a high-speed blender, and blend until smooth, and set aside.

3. Set the Instant Pot to sauté, and heat the oil. Add the onion, celery, and garlic, and cook until the onion is translucent.

4. Add the bay leaves, black pepper, paprika, 6 cups water or broth, split peas, and salt. Seal the lid, and cook at high pressure for 18 minutes.

5. Let the pressure release naturally for 15 minutes, then release manually the rest of the way.

6. Transfer the cauliflower mixture to the soup, and stir to combine.

7. Add more water as needed, to reach your desired consistency.

8. Stir in the prosciutto, if using, and adjust the seasoning as needed.

Creamy Tomato Soup

Yes, I am Dr. Gundry and I approve this tomato soup. Pressure-cooking the tomatoes takes care of the lectins; cauliflower adds gut-friendly nutrition; and garlic, basil, paprika, and oregano make this soup sing with flavor. Pair it with a slice of grilled Hearty Sandwich Bread (page 00) smeared with a little goat cheese for a Plant Paradox–approved version of grilled cheese and tomato soup!

SERVES 6

¼ cup extra-virgin olive oil

1 large onion, minced

1 pound cauliflower florets

1 teaspoon sea salt

1 teaspoon garlic powder

1 teaspoon dried oregano

½ teaspoon sweet paprika

1 teaspoon dried basil

2 28-ounce cans of peeled, seeded tomatoes (such as Italian San Marzano tomatoes)

4 cups chicken or vegetable broth

1 tablespoon lemon juice

¼ cup basil pesto, plus more for serving

Fresh basil leaves, for serving (optional)

1. Set your Instant Pot to sauté, and heat the oil.

2. Add the onion, cauliflower, salt, garlic powder, oregano, paprika, and basil, and cook, stirring occasionally, until the onion is wilted and the spices are very fragrant.

3. Then add the tomatoes, broth, lemon jiuce, and pesto and seal the pot.

4. Switch to high pressure, and cook for 15 minutes. Release the pressure with a natural release.

5. Using an immersion blender (or transfer to a high-speed blender), blend the soup until creamy.

6. Taste, and adjust the seasoning as needed.

7. Garnish with the pesto or some fresh basil leaves if using.

Ultra-Creamy Butternut Squash Soup

Butternut squash, like its cousin, pumpkin, is not typically permitted on the Plant Paradox plan. But I know how much people love this fall-favorite dish, so I wanted to find a way to recreate it. By pressure cooking the squash, adding in some resistant starch in the form of sweet potatoes, and swapping out dairy for coconut milk, I believe I've created an even more delicious and elegant version than the original!

SERVES 4 TO 6

¼ cup olive oil

2 large onions, diced

1 pound butternut squash, peeled, seeded, and chopped

1 pound sweet potatoes, peeled and chopped

3 ribs celery, diced

4 tablespoons fresh sage, minced

2 cloves garlic, minced

1 teaspoon paprika

1 teaspoon salt

½ teaspoon freshly ground black pepper

½ teaspoon nutmeg

¼ teaspoon cinnamon, plus more for garnish

2 cups cauliflower rice

1 can unsweetened coconut milk

4 cups chicken or vegetable broth

Coconut yogurt, for serving

1. Set your Instant Pot to sauté, and heat the oil.

2. Add the onions, squash, sweet potatoes, and celery, and cook, stirring occasionally, until the onions are transluscent.

3. Then add the sage, paprika, salt, black pepper, nutmeg, cinnamon, and cauliflower rice, and sauté an additional minute, stirring frequently, until fragrant.

4. Add the coconut milk and stock, and seal the pot.

5. Cook on high pressure for 10 minutes, then release pressure manually.

6. Using an immersion blender, blend until smooth, or transfer to a high-speed blender, adding water if the soup is too thick.

7. Taste, and adjust seasoning as desired.

8. Serve garnished with a sprinkle of cinnamon and a dollop of coconut yogurt.

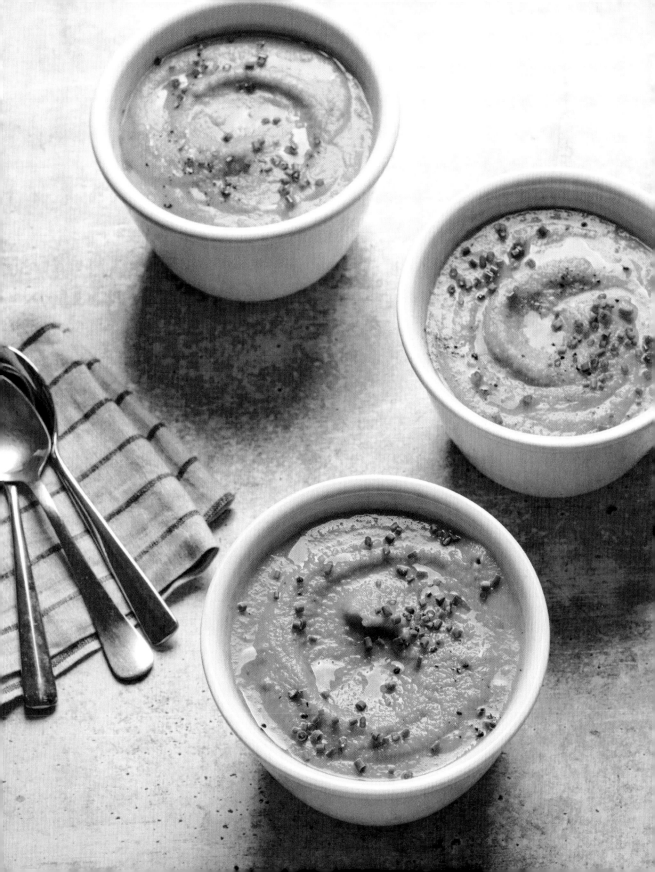

chapter nine

Lunchbox Essentials

Thanksgiving Sandwich

Thanksgiving is a marvelous opportunity to sit down with family and be grateful for the bounty in your life—and on your plate. In our household it seems like there are always plenty of leftovers, which means delicious, inventive ways to use them up. Here, I've taken my favorite Thanksgiving dinner elements and created a delicious and healthy sandwich, extending the holiday in the best possible way.

MAKES 1 SANDWICH

2 slices Sturdy Sandwich Bread (page 164)

1 to 2 slices kosher or pastured turkey (see Autumn Sheet Pan Dinner, page 118).

¼ cup Five-Minute Brussels Sprouts Salad (page 183)

¼ cup Stale Bread Stuffing (page 187)

1 tablespoon Cranberry-Orange Sauce (page 227)

1 tablespoon extra-virgin olive oil

¼ red onion, minced

1 teaspoon dried poultry seasoning

¼ ripe avocado

1. Bring the bread, turkey, Brussels sprouts, stuffing, and Cranberry-Orange Sauce to room temperature. (Chances are, you're making this because you've got leftovers in the fridge, right?)

2. In a small sauté pan, heat the olive oil over medium heat. Add the onion and poultry seasoning, and cook, stirring frequently, until the mixture is very fragrant.

3. Let cool to room temperature, then mash in the avocado.

4. Spread a thin layer of the avocado mash on each slice of bread. Layer on the Cranberry-Orange Sauce, stuffing, Brussels sprouts, and turkey.

5. Serve, and enjoy!

Sturdy Sandwich Bread

If you have a school-aged child, chances are you make a lot of sandwiches. They are a standby of packed lunches for good reason—they're easy to make, affordable, and travel well. Unfortunately, most of the bread you can buy commercially—yes, even the stuff that looks healthy—wreaks havoc on your gut. But never fear: you and your kids can have your sandwich and eat it too! The trick is making a loaf of this bread and keeping slices in the freezer for easy use. And unlike some gluten-free breads, this bread is sturdy enough to hold up to serious sandwich-making without falling apart!

MAKES 1 LOAF

¼ cup avocado oil, plus extra for greasing

2½ cups millet flour, divided, plus extra for kneading

1 cup tapioca starch

¼ cup arrowroot powder

¾ cup ground golden flaxseed

¼ cup psyllium husk flakes

½ teaspoon kosher salt

2 large omega-3 eggs, beaten

1 tablespoon raw honey, preferably local

2 cups lukewarm water (no warmer than 110ºF)

2 packets instant yeast (4½ teaspoons)

1. Prepare a 10 x 5-inch loaf pan by greasing it with avocado oil, and lining it with parchment, and set aside.

2. In a large bowl, whisk together 2 cups millet flour, the tapioca starch, arrowroot powder, flaxseed, psyllium, and salt.

3. In a small bowl, add the eggs, ¼ cup oil, honey, water, and yeast, and whisk until well combined.

4. Make a well in the dry mixture, and pour the wet mixture into the center.

5. Using a spatula, fold in the wet mixture until well combined. The dough should be cohesive, but a bit sticky/loose, and wetter than a traditional bread dough. If it feels too sticky, add the remaining millet flour, about 2 tablespoons at a time.

6. Grease a large bowl with avocado oil. Scrape the dough into the greased bowl, and oil the surface of the dough lightly. Cover with plastic wrap, and set in a warm place until the dough has doubled (about 30 minutes).

7. Lightly flour a work surface with millet flour. Punch down the dough, and knead lightly for a few minutes, then shape into a log, transfer to the prepared loaf pan, and set aside.

8. Preheat the oven to 375ºF. After the dough has rested for about 20 minutes, transfer to the oven and bake for 45 to 50 minutes.

9. Remove the pan from the oven, and let cool until you can handle the loaf.

10. Remove the loaf from the pan, and continue to allow to cool. Do not slice until completely cooled.

11. Store leftovers at room temperature for 3 to 4 days, or slice and store in the freezer for up to 3 weeks. (Just thaw in the toaster.)

The "Sandwich Salads:" Egg, Tuna, Hearts of Palm

Now that you have Sturdy Sandwich Bread (page 164), you need something to put between the slices. These delicious salads are packed with good-for-you ingredients, and they also work well over a bed of leafy greens. I suggest choosing one salad a week and making a big batch to use as needed—a true time-saver. The creaminess in these salads comes not from mayonnaise but an avocado and yogurt-based sauce, which I find much more delicious than mayo!

EACH SALAD SERVES 4

Egg Salad

4 large hard-boiled Omega-3 eggs, peeled

1 batch Salad Sauce (recipe follows)

½ teaspoon sea salt

¼ teaspoon freshly ground black pepper

½ teaspoon paprika

½ sweet onion, finely minced

½ cup finely minced jicama

¼ cup minced Italian parsley

1. Separate the hard-boiled egg whites and yolks. Finely chop the whites and place into a large bowl.

2. In a separate bowl, add the yolks and whisk in the sauce, salt, black pepper, and paprika, until a slightly chunky sauce is formed, and set aside.

3. To the egg whites, add the onion, jicama, and Italian parsley and stir to combine. Add the sauce into the egg white mixture, and fold to combine.

4. Serve on my Sturdy Sandwich Bread or over a bed of leafy greens

Salad Sauce

MAKES 1 BATCH

1 ripe avocado

1 tablespoon extra-virgin olive oil

1 tablespoon Dijon mustard

¼ cup plain goat's milk or coconut yogurt

Juice of ½ a lemon

To make in the food processor: In the work bowl of a food processor fitted with an S-blade, add the avocado, oil, mustard, yogurt, and lemon juice, and pulse until smooth and creamy.

Tuna Salad

1 can (6-ounces) wild-caught tuna, packed in water

1 batch Salad Sauce (recipe follows)

¼ cup minced celery

½ sweet onion, minced

½ cup diced jicama or ½ cup diced apple (in season, only)

½ cup toasted walnuts, chopped

¼ cup fresh parsley, minced

¼ cup fresh dill, minced

salt (optional)

1. In a large bowl, stir together the tuna and sauce until well combined.

2. Fold in the celery, onion, jicama, and walnuts until well combined.

3. Add the parsley and dill, and fold gently, so as not to bruise the herbs.

4. Taste, and add a little salt, if you'd like.

5. Serve on my Sturdy Sandwich Bread or over a bed of leafy greens.

Hearts of Palm Salad

6 ounces canned hearts of palm, finely chopped

1 batch Salad Sauce (recipe follows)

¼ cup minced celery

½ sweet onion, minced

½ cup toasted walnuts, chopped

¼ cup fresh parsley, minced

¼ cup fresh dill, minced

Juice of ½ a lemon

salt (optional)

1. In a large bowl, stir together the hearts of palm and sauce until well combined.

2. Fold in the celery, onion, and walnuts until well combined.

3. Add the parsley, dill, and lemon juice and fold gently, so as not to bruise the herbs.

4. Taste, and add a little salt, if you'd like.

5. Serve on my Sturdy Sandwich Bread or over a bed of leafy greens.

To make by hand: In a bowl, mash the avocado until smooth, then add the oil, mustard, yogurt, and lemon juice, and stir until smooth.

Before using: In a bowl, whisk the avocado mixture until "fluffy," for about 1 to 2 minutes.

Bonus tip: Kids *love* whisking stuff, so get the whole family involved!

Vegetable Roll-Ups

Just about every kid I know, no matter how picky, will eat a roll-up. Unfortunately, the roll-ups wrapped in store-bought tortillas are lectin-packed carb bombs that aren't going to give your kids the energy and brainpower they need to get through the school day. With these reinvented roll-ups, your kids can enjoy a lunchtime favorite and a happy tummy all afternoon.

SERVES 1

2 large collard greens leaves

1 tablespoon extra-virgin olive oil

¼ cup minced mushrooms

¼ white onion, finely chopped

¼ cup shredded Brussels sprouts

½ ripe avocado

¼ teaspoon sea salt

Zest and juice of 1 lemon

¼ cup Lectin-Light Hummus (page 216)

1. Carefully remove the stems from the collard greens, leaving as much of the leaves intact as possible, and set aside.

2. In a large sauté pan, heat the oil over medium high. Add the mushrooms and onion and sauté, stirring occasionally, until the onion is translucent. Add the Brussels sprouts, and continue to cook until the sprouts smell nutty and delicious.

3. Remove from the heat and let cool to room temperature.

4. Meanwhile, in a bowl, mash together the avocado, salt, lemon juice, and lemon zest. Fold into the cooled sprouts mixture, and set aside.

5. Spread each prepared collard green leaf with a bit of hummus, and add the Brussels sprout mixture. Roll like a burrito, and serve. You can also cut these sushi style before adding to a lunchbox.

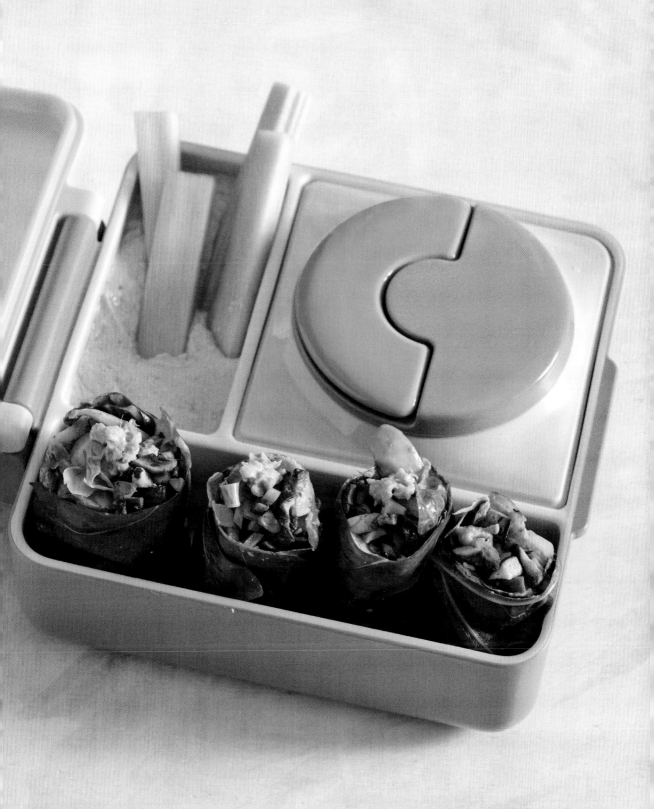

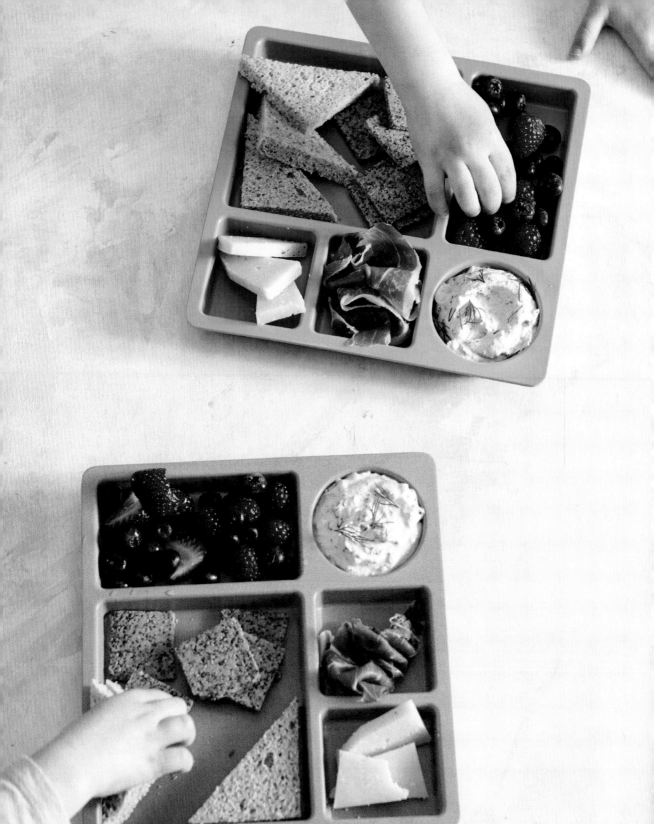

Lectin-Free Lunch Kits

When prepackaged lunch-assembly kits hit the scene, they were all the rage with kids in school, traded around cafeterias like currency. As you probably suspect, these cute, ready-to-eat meals are filled with nasty preservatives and chemicals—not to mention, plenty of lectins. Plus, they're packed in single-use plastic, which not only imparts BPA (a well-known endocrine disruptor), but also pollutes our planet. My lunch kits are a play on this cult classic, but without any of the gut-inflaming lectins. Best of all, they are delicious.

SERVES 1

For the Lunch Kits:

4 to 5 Cheesy Almond Crackers (page 172)

¼ cup Garlic and Chive "Cheese" Spread (page 173)

1 to 2 ounces Plant Paradox–approved meat or cheese, sliced*

1 large leaf lettuce, torn into 4 to 5 pieces

¼ cup in-season fruit, cut into bite-size pieces.

1. To assemble your lunch box, pack the crackers, "cheese" spread, meat, lettuce, and fruit in a divided container. You can use multiple small containers, a bento-box style carrier, or even a shallow Tupperware piece fitted with muffin-liners as dividers. (If you do the latter, I suggest stashing the fruit separately.)

2. When ready to eat, layer the crackers with a smear of "cheese" spread, the lettuce, and the meat. Eat with the fruit on the side.

If your child prefers cured meat, try prosciutto. You can also use sliced roast turkey or pastured chicken, or even wild-caught salmon. For cheese, stick to aged, Southern European cheeses, and sheep's and goat's milk cheese whenever possible.

Cheesy Almond Crackers

MAKES 20 TO 30 CRACKERS

1¾ cups almond flour

¼ cup grated Parmigiano-Reggiano or nutritional yeast

1 large omega-3 egg or one flax egg*

¼ cup lightly toasted white sesame seeds

¼ cup poppy seeds

1 tablespoon coconut oil or grass-fed French or Italian butter

½ teaspoon ground turmeric

½ teaspoon sea salt

½ teaspoon ground garlic

½ teaspoon fresh minced rosemary

¼ teaspoon ground freshly ground black pepper

To make a flax egg, combine 1 tablespoon organic ground flaxseeds with 3 tablespoons water. Let sit for at least 5 minutes.

1. Preheat the oven to 350°F. Line a rimmed baking sheet with parchment, and set aside.

2. In a large bowl, add all ingredients and stir until well combined. The mixture should be smooth and crumbly, but hold together when you form it into a ball.

3. Place the cracker dough onto the prepared baking sheet, flatten into a rough square shape, and top with a second piece of parchment.

4. Roll the dough into a thin rectangle, approximately the size of a sheet of paper (8 x 11 inches). Remove top layer of parchment, and cut the dough into small cracker-size squares.

5. Bake for 15 to 20 minutes, keeping an eye on the crackers so they don't burn.

6. Remove the baking sheet from oven, flip the crackers over, and bake an additional 10 to 15 minutes.

7. Remove from the oven, and let cool to room temperature before using. Store extra crackers in an airtight container for 1–2 days.

Garlic and Chive "Cheese" Spread

MAKES 1½ CUPS

2 cups chopped macadamia nuts, soaked in water 2 to 4 hours, then drained

½ cup water

Juice of 1 lemon

Finely grated zest of 1 lemon

½ cup nutritional yeast

1 teaspoon smoked paprika

1 to 2 cloves garlic, peeled and chopped

¼ cup finely chopped chives

¼ cup finely chopped Italian parsley

Sea salt to taste

1. In a high-speed blender or the bowl of a food processor fitted with an S-blade, add the drained nuts, water, lemon juice, and lemon zest and pulse until combined, then blend until very smooth.

2. Add the nutritional yeast, paprika, and garlic and blend until smooth and well combined.

3. Transfer the mixture to a bowl and fold in the chives and parsley, along with salt to taste, then serve. Store in an airtight container in the refrigerator for up to 1 week.

Kids' Mediterranean Platter

When "Lectin Free Mama" and blogger Autumn Boyle makes lunch for her three-year-old daughter, she almost always packs a deconstructed version of the meals she and her husband eat (like this riff on a Greek salad). That way, her daughter has a chance to explore each ingredient individually. Her best "kid feeding" advice is to stretch out your mealtimes as long as possible—because the longer your child stays at the table, the longer they will have to try everything on their plate.

SERVES 4

1 bunch asparagus, ends trimmed, and broken in half

1 cup pressure-cooked chickpeas or Eden brand, drained and rinsed

½ teaspoon ground cumin

Salt and pepper to taste

Juice of ½ a lemon

1 tablespoon tahini

1 clove garlic, finely minced

¼ cup extra-virgin olive oil

4 Perfect Pressure Cooker Hard-Boiled Eggs (page 235), peeled and quartered

1 pint fresh figs, halved

1 bunch radishes, chopped

½ cup pitted olives

½ cup crumbled sheep's or goat's milk feta

2 Romaine lettuce hearts, leaves separated

1. Bring a pot of water to a boil and add the asparagus. Cook approximately 3 minutes, until the asparagus is bright green and crisp-tender.

2. Transfer the asparagus to a bowl of very cold (or ice) water.

3. In a small bowl, combine the chickpeas, cumin, and a pinch of both the salt and the pepper, and set aside.

4. In a separate small bowl, whisk together the lemon juice, tahini, garlic, 1 tablespoon water, and a small pinch of salt.

5. Slowly drizzle in the oil, stirring to create a creamy dressing, and set aside.

6. Serve the asparagus, chickpeas, and eggs with the figs, radishes, olives, and feta over the lettuce leaves, either as a salad, or keeping separate in a bento box, so your child can customize their meal.

Avocado and Cheddar Sweet Potato Toasts

Avocado toast seems to have taken the world (or at least, Instagram) by storm, but many versions of this "healthy meal" you'll find posted on social media are actually far from healthy. I love this twist on the trendy dish, created again by "Lectin Free Mama" Autum Boyle, who swaps in resistant starch-rich sweet potatoes for lectin-filled bread. The addition of a little goat's milk cheddar gives these "toasts" even more kid appeal.

SERVES 4

2 large sweet potatoes, sliced lengthwise into ½-inch-thick slabs

1 tablespoon avocado oil

½ teaspoon sea salt

½ teaspoon freshly ground black pepper

2 avocados, thinly sliced*

4 radishes, thinly sliced

2 ounces goat's milk Cheddar, shredded

Juice of 1 lime

Broccoli sprouts, for serving

1. Preheat the oven to 450°F.

2. Coat each sweet potato with the oil and sprinkle generously with the salt and pepper. Spread on a baking sheet and roast for 15 minutes, flipping halfway through, until tender and slightly brown.

3. Use immediately, or chill overnight.

4. Divide the avocados, radishes, and Cheddar among the sweet potato "toasts."

5. Sprinkle the lime juice over the "toasts," and top with the broccoli sprouts.

If packing in a lunch box, consider using prepackaged tomato-free guacamole, or mash the avocado with lime juice to prevent excessive browning.

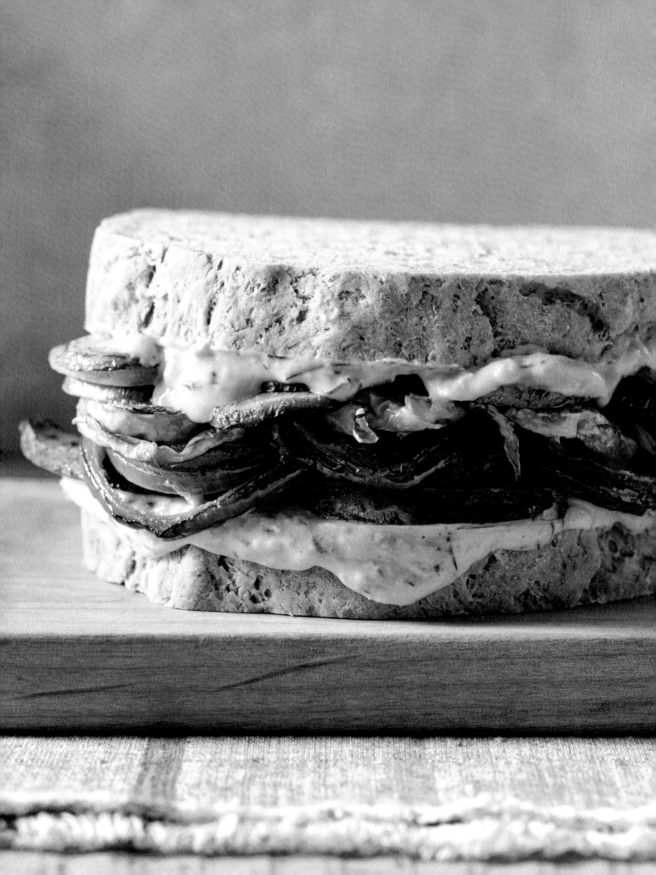

Ultimate Roast Vegetable Sandwich

This vegetarian sandwich is crowd-pleasing combo of subtle flavors that delights kids and adults alike. And with a healthy serving of hummus, you're getting in a nice hit of plant-based protein in addition to all of the delicious roasted vegetables. The true star of the show, however, might be the creamy Tangy Ranch Dressing/Dip—it takes your typical veggie sandwich up several notches. Beware—it is addicting!

SERVES 2

2 tablespoons Lectin-Light Hummus (page 216)

2 tablespoons Tangy Ranch Dressing/Dip (page 219)

2 tablespoons extra-virgin olive oil

1 tablespoon minced fresh rosemary

½ teaspoon fine sea salt

1 portobello mushroom cap, thinly sliced

¼ cup thinly sliced radishes

½ cup thinly sliced Brussels sprouts

½ onion or 2 shallots, thinly sliced

4 slices Sturdy Sandwich Bread (page 164) or another lectin-free sandwich bread

1. Preheat the oven to 425°F.

2. In a small bowl, combine the hummus and ranch dressing. Refrigerate until needed.

3. In another bowl, toss together the olive oil, rosemary, salt, mushroom cap, radishes, Brussels sprouts, and onion.

4. Spread the vegetables on a rimmed baking sheet, and bake for 15 to 20 minutes, until tender.

5. Remove from the oven, and let cool to room temperature.

6. Toast the bread lightly, then spread each slice liberally with the hummus mixture.

7. Layer the vegetables on top of the hummus, close the sandwich, and enjoy.

Lettuce Wrap "Tacos"

Who doesn't love a taco? Kids are always happy to eat with their hands, and I've never met a grownup who isn't up for getting his or her hands dirty in the name of a great taco. While tacos can be a healthy choice, the tortilla wrapper—whether corn or flour—is loaded with lectins. Here, I've swapped out the traditional wrapper for crunchy lettuce leaves and filled them with veggies and protein for a gut-friendly, nutrition-packed taco party. For a vegetarian option, you can use jackfruit that has been canned in brine, or frozen.

SERVES 4

¼ cup extra-virgin olive oil

½ onion, minced

2 cups finely minced kale

4 cloves garlic, minced

1 bag Quorn crumbles, 2 cups shredded leftover chicken, or 2 cups shredded jackfruit

½ teaspoon cumin

½ teaspoon sweet paprika

½ teaspoon freshly ground black pepper

½ teaspoon fine sea salt

Finely grated zest of 1 orange

½ cup chicken or vegetable broth

1 head butter lettuce, leaves separated from core

1 avocado, peeled, pitted, and sliced

¼ cup minced fresh cilantro

½ cup Spicy Tomato Salsa (page 000)

1. In a large sauté pan, heat the oil over medium heat. Add the onion and sauté 2 to 3 minutes, until the onion becomes translucent.

2. Add the kale, garlic, and protein of your choice and continue to cook until the kale is wilted, the garlic is fragrant, and the mixture is heated through.

3. Add the cumin, paprika, black pepper, salt, and orange zest and sauté for 2 to 3 minutes, until very fragrant.

4. Then add the broth, reduce the heat to low, and simmer until the broth has reduced by half. Use the filling immediately, or refrigerate for later (it's great at room temperature!)

5. To assemble the tacos, add some of the filling to each lettuce leaf. Top with the avocado, cilantro, and salsa before serving.

6. To pack in a lunchbox, pack each component separately for your little one to assemble. I suggest squeezing some lime juice on the avocado to keep it from turning brown.

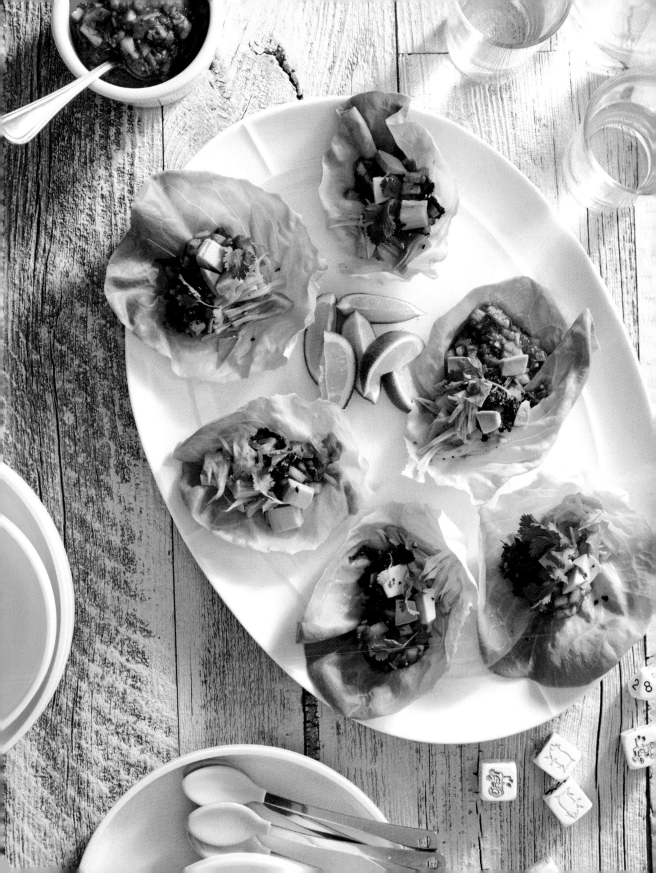

chapter ten

Sensational Sides

Buttery Mashed Cauliflower

Cauliflower is a nutritional powerhouse and easily stands in anywhere potatoes typically take the leading role. Here, it replaces potatoes in a mash that is velvety and luscious. This mash makes a great accompaniment to my Perfect Roasted Chicken (page 00) or my Braised Chicken with Artichokes (page 00). If serving simply, feel free to top with a small dollop of organic sour cream and some chives, if you like.

SERVES 4

¼ cup extra-virgin olive oil or grass-fed butter

4 cloves garlic, smashed

1 large cauliflower, florets only (about 5 cups)

1½ cups chicken or vegetable broth

½ teaspoon sea salt

½ cup grated Parmigiano-Reggiano (optional)

1. Set your Instant Pot to sauté, and heat the oil.

2. Add the garlic, and sauté until fragrant.

3. Then add the cauliflower, broth, and salt, and seal the pot. Cook on high pressure for 5 minutes, then release the pressure with a quick release.

4. Let the cauliflower rest for 3 minutes.

5. Strain the excess liquid into a bowl, and transfer the cauliflower and garlic to the bowl of a food processor fitted with an S-blade or do this in a bowl with a potato masher.

6. Add the Parmigiano-Reggiano, if using, and process or mash until smooth and creamy.

7. Taste, add salt as needed, and serve.

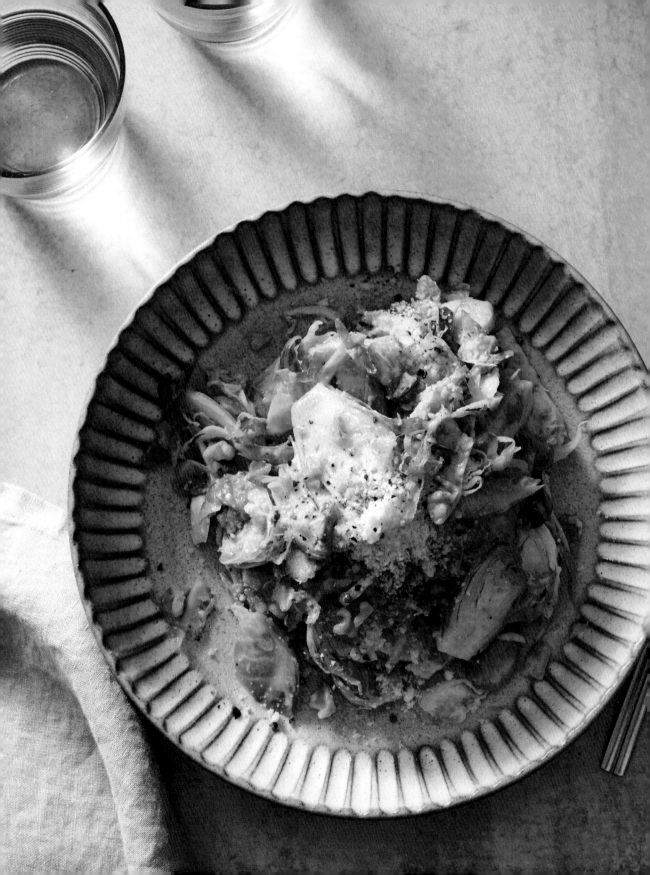

Five-Minute Brussels Sprouts Salad

The name says it all—this flavorful salad takes only five minutes to put together. A zesty dressing made with lemon juice, olive oil, and mustard highlights the earthy notes of the sprouts. Finish it all off with a sprinkle of walnuts for those all-important omega-3s and some crunch.

SERVES 4

1 pound shredded Brussels sprouts (pre-bagged, shredded in a food processor, or shaved on a mandoline)

Zest and juice of 1 lemon

½ teaspoon sea salt

½ teaspoon freshly ground black pepper

2 tablespoons extra-virgin olive oil

1 teaspoon Dijon mustard

¼ cup pecorino Romano or nutritional yeast

¼ cup toasted walnuts

1. In a large bowl, combine the Brussels sprouts, lemon zest, and salt.

2. Massage with your fingertips until the sprouts are bright green and tender.

3. In a separate bowl, whisk together the lemon juice, pepper, oil, and mustard until smooth.

4. Toss the with Brussels sprouts, cheese or nutritional yeast, and walnuts before serving.

Keto Naan Bread

Naan is a popular bread in Northern Indian cuisine that is delicious on its own, or served as a side with a soup or stew. While most naan is made from wheat, this Plant Paradox–compliant, keto-friendly version is made with coconut flour but still uses traditional spices—minced garlic and cumin—to ensure it tastes like the original.

SERVES 6 TO 8

¾ cup coconut flour

2 tablespoons ground psyllium husk powder

½ teaspoon garlic powder

½ teaspoon baking powder

¼ teaspoon cumin

1 teaspoon sea salt

4 tablespoons avocado oil

1 to 2 cups boiling water

2 tablespoons minced garlic

Minced cilantro, for serving

1. Preheat the oven to 350°F. Line a rimmed baking sheet with parchment, and set aside. (You can also do this in a sauté pan, but the naan holds together better in the oven.)

2. In a large bowl, mix together the flour, psyllium husk powder, garlic powder, baking powder, cumin, and salt.

3. Add the oil and 1 cup water and stir until the dough is cohesive. Add more water, bit by bit, until the dough comes together.

4. Let rest for 5 minutes for the dough to hydrate. The dough should be the consistency of Play-Doh—if too thin, add more psyllium husk, if too thick, add more water, a tiny bit at a time. (Your kids will love playing with the dough.)

5. Divide the dough into 6 to 8 balls, depending on how many people you're serving. Flatten each dough ball with your hands, and pat the minced garlic onto the top of each one.

6. Bake until the naan is golden brown, and the garlic is fragrant. If cooking in a skillet, fry in coconut oil until golden brown.

7. Sprinkle with the cilantro and serve with any of the curries or stews in this book.

Quick Baguette

Is there *anything* more delicious than a fresh loaf of bread, hot from the oven? Especially if it's a crispy, chewy baguette? This recipe, from "Lectin Free Gourmet" creator Kristine Anderson Wylie, uses buffalo mozzarella to replace the stretch and texture traditionally provided by gluten. Use slices of this bread in the French toast recipes on page 94–95, or simply dip it in olive oil and enjoy!

MAKES 2 BAGUETTES

100% olive oil cooking spray

3 large omega-3 eggs

½ cup A2 milk or coconut milk

1 cup grated buffalo mozzarella

2 tablespoons extra-virgin olive oil

1 teaspoon sea salt

1½ cups cassava flour

1½ cups tapioca starch

1. Preheat the oven to 485°F (475°F will work too). Line a sheet tray with parchment or spray a baguette pan with oil, and set aside.

2. In a stand mixer fitted with a whisk attachment, whip the eggs until extremely frothy, about 3 minutes.

3. Switch the whisk attachment for the dough hook, and add the milk, mozzarella, oil, and salt the to mixer and blend together well.

4. In a separate bowl, combine the cassava and tapioca flours.

5. With the mixer on low, gradually add the flour until a dough ball forms. It should be the consistency of regular bread dough. If too thick, add water, a teaspoon at a time. If too loose, add more flour.

6. Divide the dough ball in half. Roll each half into a 12-inch baguette, and arrange on the prepared sheet pan or in the baguette pan.

7. Score each baguette with ¼-inch-deep diagonal cuts across the top.

8. Bake for 22 to 25 minutes until the baguettes are a rich golden brown, puffy, and crusty. (If you had to set your oven at 475°F, bake for 25 to 30 minutes.)

Crowd-Pleasing Zucchini and Onions

Cooking zucchini in a pressure cooker eliminates the harmful lectins and results in a side that is delicious, nourishing, and is a great accompaniment to a number of main courses. Try to use baby zucchini if you can find it, which has fewer seeds. This dish pairs well with my Portobello "Pot Roast" (page 140) or BBQ Pulled Pork (page 145).

SERVES 4 TO 6

¼ cup extra-virgin olive oil

1 large yellow onion, thinly sliced

4 cups thinly sliced peeled baby zucchini

2 cups thinly sliced celery

1 ½ cups chicken or vegetable broth

1 tablespoon dried basil

½ teaspoon freshly ground black pepper

½ teaspoon sea salt

1. Set your Instant Pot to sauté, and heat the oil.

2. Add the onion, and sauté until the onion begins to brown.

3. Then add the zucchini, celery, chicken broth, basil, pepper, and sea salt. Seal the pot, and cook on high pressure for 3 to 4 minutes.

4. Release the pressure with a quick release.

5. Serve, and enjoy.

Stale Bread Stuffing

You heard it here first: You can enjoy a traditional holiday stuffing on the Plant Paradox plan! All you need is a loaf of Sturdy Sandwich Bread that's a few days old and some basic pantry ingredients to create a bread stuffing that tastes like home. I love the flavor and aroma of fresh thyme and sage, but you can add in any of your favorite herbs and spices.

SERVES 4 TO 6

⅓ cup extra-virgin olive oil

1 large onion, minced

5 ribs celery, minced

3 cups mushrooms, minced

4 cloves garlic, minced

2 tablespoons minced fresh sage

1 tablespoon fresh thyme leaves

1 tablespoon poultry seasoning

1 teaspoon sweet paprika

1 teaspoon sea salt

1 teaspoon freshly ground black pepper

3 cups cubed stale Sturdy Sandwich Bread (page 164)

1 to 2 cups chicken or vegetable broth

1. Preheat the oven to 350°F.

2. In a large oven-safe skillet over medium high, heat the oil.

3. Add the onion, celery, and mushrooms, and cook, stirring occasionally, until the vegetables are tender.

4. Add the garlic, sage, thyme, poultry seasoning, paprika, salt, black pepper, and cubed bread, and sauté until the mixture is very fragrant.

5. Remove from the heat and drizzle in the broth until the mixture is very moist.

6. Transfer to the oven and bake for 15 to 20 minutes, until the top is crispy.

7. Serve, and enjoy.

Mushroom Fries

Hearty, flavorful, and polyphenol-rich portobellos have just the right texture to stand in for potatoes in my "fries," which are perfect for oven baking or air frying. This umami-rich side isn't just for kids—if you have anyone in your family who's a fan of "truffle fries," it's safe to say they'll be a fan of these 'shroom fries as well!

SERVES 4 AS A SIDE

2 large omega-3 eggs

1 cup almond flour

¼ cup flaxseed meal

⅔ cup grated Parmigiano-Reggiano or nutritional yeast

½ teaspoon garlic powder

½ teaspoon cumin

½ teaspoon sweet paprika

4 portobello mushroom caps, gills removed, sliced ¼-inch thick

1 teaspoon sea salt

1. In a small bowl, whisk together the eggs with a small splash of water, and set aside.

2. In another bowl, combine the almond flour, flaxseed meal, Parmigiano-Reggiano or nutritional yeast, garlic powder, cumin, and paprika. DO NOT add the salt at this point.

3. Dip each piece of the mushrooms in the eggs, then roll in the almond flour mixture, coating evenly. Set on a rimmed baking sheet in a single layer.

4. Cook the mushroom fries using one of the two following methods:

TO COOK IN THE OVEN:

1. Place a rimmed baking sheet in a cold oven, and preheat the oven (and baking sheet) to 400°F.

2. When hot, thoroughly grease the baking sheet with oil, then carefully arrange the mushrooms in a single layer on the tray.

3. Bake for 10 to12 minutes, then flip, and bake for an additional 5 to 6 minutes.

4. Sprinkle with the salt before serving.

1. Preheat the air fryer to 350ºF.

2. Carefully grease the fryer basket with cooking spray, and arrange the mushrooms in a single layer in the basket. You may need to cook in batches.

3. Cook for 12 minutes, flipping halfway through.

4. Remove the fries from the basket and sprinkle with the salt before serving.

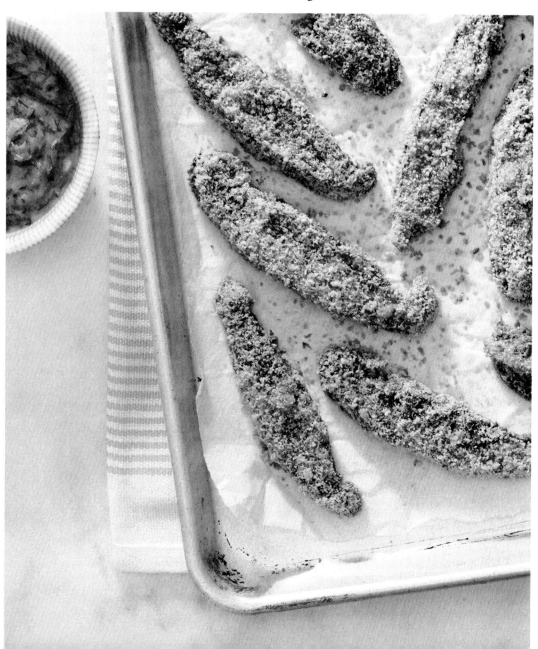

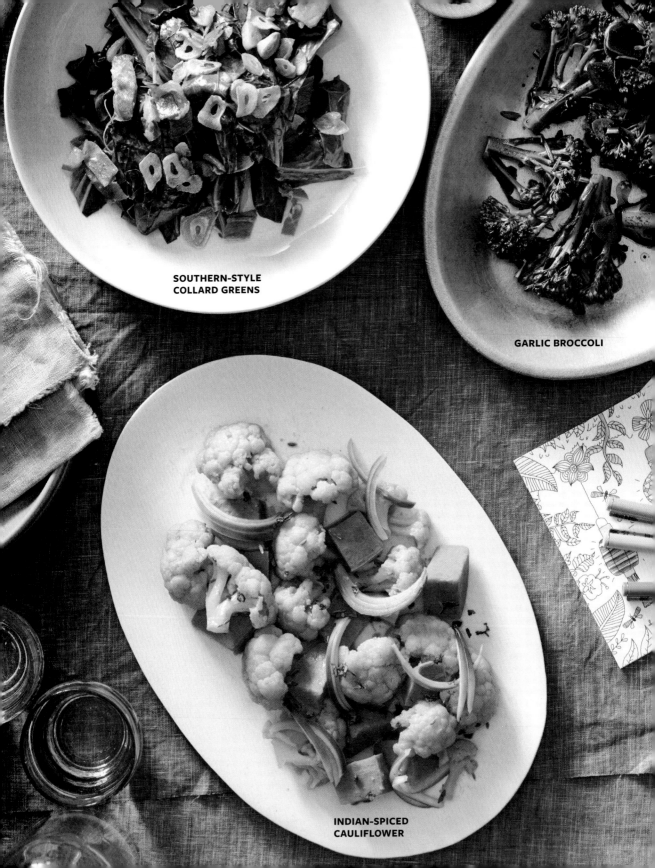

SOUTHERN-STYLE COLLARD GREENS

GARLIC BROCCOLI

INDIAN-SPICED CAULIFLOWER

Indian-Spiced Cauliflower

While cauliflower is used throughout this book as a stand-in for white potatoes and other lectin-rich foods, here it finally gets its moment in the spotlight. Enhanced with Indian spices such as garam masala and anti-inflammatory turmeric, this dish pairs nicely with my Keto Naan Bread (page 184).

SERVES 4

1 tablespoon avocado oil

½ teaspoon whole cumin seeds

1 large red onion, minced

1 teaspoon grated fresh ginger

2 cloves garlic, finely grated

1 teaspoon coriander

1 teaspoon turmeric

½ teaspoon garam masala

½ teaspoon sea salt

⅓ cup water

2 sweet potatoes, peeled and chopped into medium pieces

1 head cauliflower, cut into large florets

2 tablespoons cilantro

1. Set your Instant Pot to sauté, and add the oil and cumin seeds. Toast the seeds until they release their fragrance.

2. Then add the onion, and cook 2 to 3 minutes until the onion is translucent.

3. Add the ginger, garlic, coriander, turmeric, garam masala, and salt, and continue to cook, stirring frequently, until fragrant.

4. Deglaze the pot with the water, and add the sweet potatoes and cauliflower, and stir.

5. Seal the pot, switch to high pressure, and let cook for 1 minute, to combine.

6. Strain off any extra water, or switch back to sauté and cook off the water.

7. Sprinkle with the cilantro before serving.

Garlic Broccoli

This is an incredibly simple but delicious side dish that pairs perfectly with any number of mains or lunches, such as Tahini-Miso Tempeh (page 126) or Pastured Chicken Nuggets (page 106). Adding balsamic vinegar gives the broccoli and the aromatics a nice hit of acid and balances the flavors.

SERVES 4

100% olive oil cooking spray

¼ cup extra-virgin olive oil

3 cloves garlic, minced

1 shallot, minced

2 tablespoons minced rosemary

1 teaspoon sea salt

5 cups broccoli florets

¼ cup balsamic vinegar

1. Preheat the oven to 450°F. Spray a rimmed baking sheet with oil, and set aside.

2. In a small bowl, stir together the oil, garlic, shallot, rosemary, and salt.

3. In another bowl, add the broccoli and pour the oil mixture over the broccoli, and toss to combine.

4. Spread into a single layer on the prepared baking sheet, and transfer to the oven.

5. Bake for 10 to 15 minutes, tossing occasionally, until the broccoli is charred on the edges and tender in the center.

6. Remove from the oven and drizzle with the vinegar before serving.

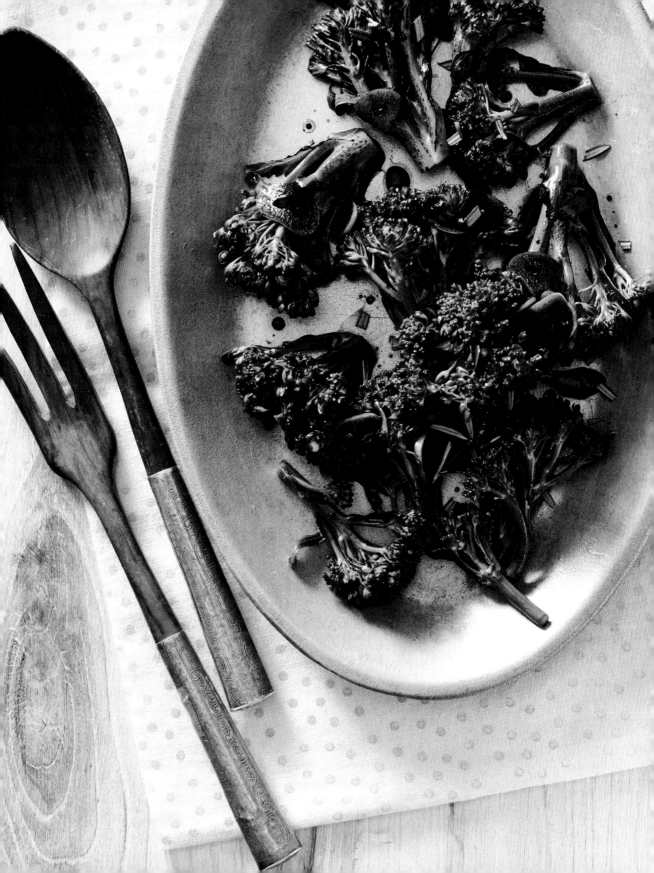

Southern-Style Collard Greens

Collard greens are a staple in the South, and often the "pot likker" (the cooking liquid in which the collards simmer) can be savored on its own as a broth. Cooking collards the old-fashioned way can take several hours, but using a pressure cooker shrinks the cook time considerably. To mimic the traditional Southern dish, add prosciutto, but feel free to skip it if you are vegetarian or vegan.

MAKES 4 ¾ CUP SERVINGS

4 tablespoons avocado oil

6 cloves garlic, thinly sliced

¼ cup minced prosciutto (optional)

½ cup red wine vinegar

¼ cup water

¼ cup monk fruit sweetener

½ cup chicken or vegetable broth

1 teaspoon paprika

1 teaspoon garlic powder

1 teaspoon freshly ground black pepper

½ teaspoon sea salt

½ teaspoon dried oregano

10 cups torn collard greens leaves, approximately 2 10-ounce bags prepared collards

1. Set your Instant Pot to sauté.

2. Add the avocado oil, garlic, and prosciutto, if using, and cook, stirring occasionally, until the garlic is fragrant.

3. Then add the vinegar, water, sweetener, broth, paprika, garlic powder, pepper, salt, oregano, and collard greens, and sauté for an additional 3 to 5 minutes, to draw any liquid out of the collard greens.

4. Switch the pot to pressure cook, seal, and cook for 25 minutes.

5. Naturally release the pressure for 10 minutes, then manually release the rest of the way.

6. Remove the lid, and sauté off any liquid you do not want (some people enjoy the braising liquid, others don't).

7. Serve, and enjoy.

Instant Pot Okra

Okra is one of those polarizing vegetables people seem to either love or hate—I am in the former camp, especially now that I have this quick, easy recipe at my fingertips. Anti-inflammatory spices cumin and turmeric add great flavor and turn the cooking liquid a beautiful golden yellow, but beware if you have white countertops—it stains!

SERVES 4

¼ cup extra-virgin olive oil

½ teaspoon cumin seeds

1 onion, sliced small

3 cloves garlic, thinly sliced

¼ teaspoon ground turmeric

½ teaspoon coriander

Zest of 1 lemon

1 teaspoon sea salt

1 pound okra, cut into ½-inch pieces

1. Set your Instant Pot to sauté, and heat about a tablespoon of the oil.

2. Add the cumin, onion, and garlic, and sauté until tender.

3. Add the turmeric, coriander, lemon zest, salt, and okra, and stir to combine.

4. Switch the Instant Pot to pressure cook, and cook for 2 minutes at low pressure (the pot may not seal).

5. Release the pressure with a quick release, and switch to sauté to cook off any excess liquid.

6. When the pot is dry, add the remaining oil and cook until the okra begins to crisp.

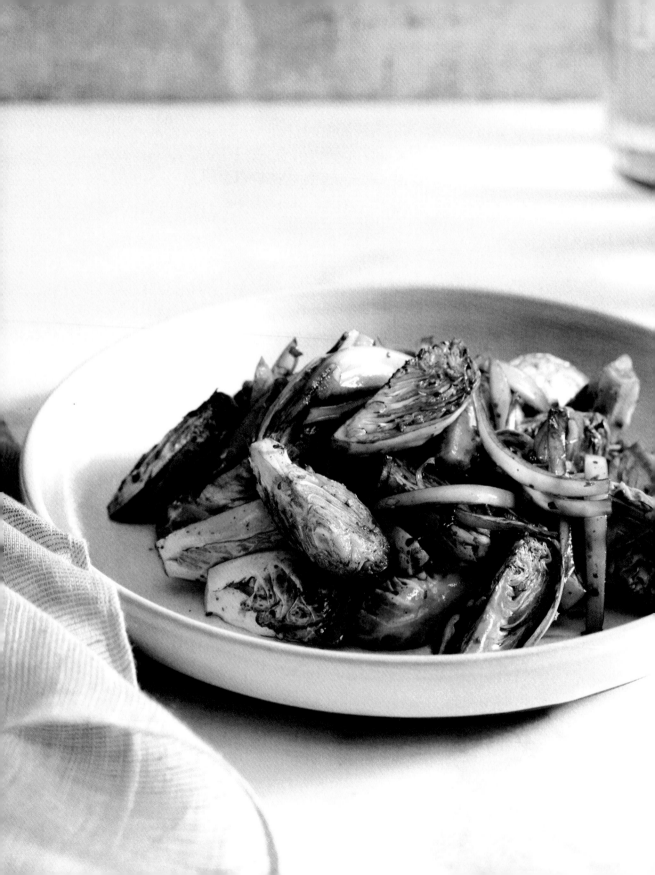

Sweet and Salty Brussels Sprouts

This recipe, as the name suggests, combines sweet and the salty flavors to create a dressing so addictive, you'll find you don't have to beg your kids to eat their Brussels sprouts! Be sure to slice your shallots paper-thin, so they will crisp up during roasting and add crunch to the final dish.

SERVES 4

¼ cup extra-virgin olive oil

4 cloves garlic, minced

1 teaspoon salt

1 teaspoon freshly ground black pepper

¼ cup balsamic vinegar

2 tablespoons yacon syrup or monk fruit sweetener

1½ pounds Brussels sprouts, quartered

1 cup thinly sliced shallots

1. Preheat the oven to 425°F.

2. In a large bowl, toss all of the ingredients until well combined.

3. Transfer the Brussels sprouts mixture to a rimmed baking sheet, and bake for 5 minutes.

4. Toss, and cook for an additional 3 to 6 minutes, until the sprouts are tender in the center and brown at the edges.

5. Serve, and enjoy.

Braised Sweet-and-Sour Cabbage

Cabbage, once regarded as undesirable peasant food, is gaining popularity these days as a humble, do-it-all and healthy ingredient. In this dish, cabbage gets a lift from caraway seeds and a generous splash of red wine vinegar, and a gentle simmer in the Instant Pot makes a delicious, delicate side that will be devoured by the whole family.

SERVES 4-6

2 tablespoons avocado oil

2 tablespoons monk fruit sweetener

1 teaspoon caraway seeds

1 small red onion, minced

1 red cabbage, finely shredded

1 cup water

Sea salt to taste

3 to 4 tablespoons red wine vinegar, to taste

1. Set your Instant Pot to sauté. Add the avocado oil, sweetener, and caraway seeds, and cook, stirring occasionally, until the seeds are fragrant.

2. Add the onion, and continue to sauté, stirring frequently, until the onion is translucent.

3. Then add the cabbage, water, and a pinch of salt.

4. Seal the pot, and cook at high pressure for 5 minutes.

5. Let pressure release naturally for 10 minutes, then manually release it the rest of the way.

6. Add the vinegar and mix well. Serve as is, or if there's too much liquid, switch to the sauté setting and cook off the extra liquid, before serving. This is best served warm.

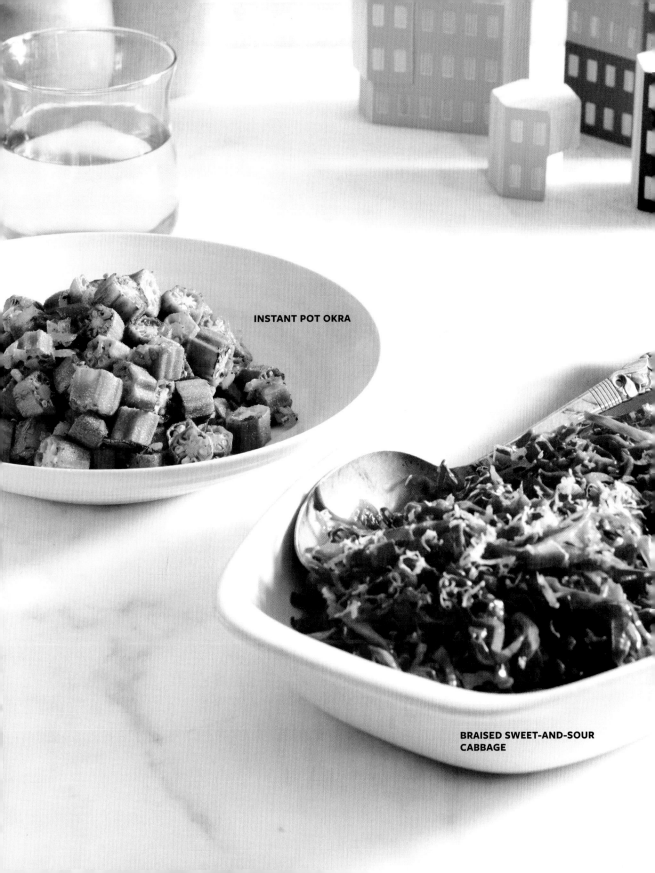

INSTANT POT OKRA

BRAISED SWEET-AND-SOUR CABBAGE

chapter eleven

Sweet
Treats

Chocolate Lava Cake

This cake is one of those back-pocket recipes you can rely on anytime company unexpectedly stays for dinner, or just when you're in the mood for a little something sweet. All you need is a handful of basic pantry ingredients and a few minutes of microwave cook time and voila—you've got an ooey-gooey molten chocolate cake!

SERVES 1

1 large omega-3 egg

1 tablespoon grass-fed butter or coconut oil, melted

1 tablespoon coconut cream

½ teaspoon vanilla extract

2 tablespoons Swerve

2 tablespoons natural cocoa powder

1 teaspoon almond flour

⅛ teaspoon baking soda

Tiny pinch of salt

100% avocado oil spray

1. In a small bowl, vigorously whisk together the egg, butter, coconut cream, and extract until the mixture lightens. (This is a great place to get kids involved.)

2. Add the Swerve, cocoa powder, almond flour, baking soda, and salt, and whisk to combine.

3. Spray a microwave-safe mug with avocado oil spray, and pour the batter into the mug.

4. Microwave for 30 to 45 seconds, so the cake is slightly firm, while the middle is not yet set.

5. If not set enough, continue to microwave at 5 to 10-second intervals until you have the consistency of a Chocolate Lava Cake.

6. Serve, and enjoy.

Macadamia Butter Chocolate Cheesecake

Forget about the tried and true combo of peanut butter and milk chocolate: This amazing cheesecake made with macadamia nuts and bittersweet chocolate will become your family's new favorite. Almond flour and cocoa powder work beautifully in the crust, and the filling, made with pureed macadamia nuts and coconut cream, is delectable.

SERVES 12

FOR THE CRUST:

1¾ cups blanched almond flour

4 tablespoons cocoa powder

3 tablespoons monk fruit sweetener

⅓ cup coconut oil or grass-fed butter

1 teaspoon vanilla extract

FOR THE FILLING:

1⅔ cups raw macadamia nuts, soaked in water overnight (or longer)

¾ cup canned unsweetened coconut cream

½ cup powdered Swerve

½ cup melted bittersweet chocolate

½ cup melted coconut oil or grass-fed butter

½ teaspoon vanilla extract

1 tablespoon almond extract

1. Preheat the oven to 375°F. Line an 8-inch springform pan with parchment, and set aside.

2. To make the crust, in the bowl of a food processor fitted with an S-blade, add the flour, cocoa powder, sweetener, coconut oil, and extract, and pulse until they come together into a smooth dough.

3. Press the dough into the base of the prepared pan, and bake for 10 to 15 minutes, until set and firm to the touch. Let cool to room temperature.

4. Meanwhile, to make the filling, in the bowl of a food processor fitted with an S-blade, add the drained nuts and coconut cream and pulse until a smooth paste is formed. Add the Swerve and continue to pulse until creamy.

5. Add the chocolate, coconut oil, and vanilla and almond extracts, and pulse until smooth. If the mixture becomes too thick, add a few tablespoons of coconut milk to thin it, then transfer to the prepared crust.

6. Place in the refrigerator and chill for at least 4 hours or until set.

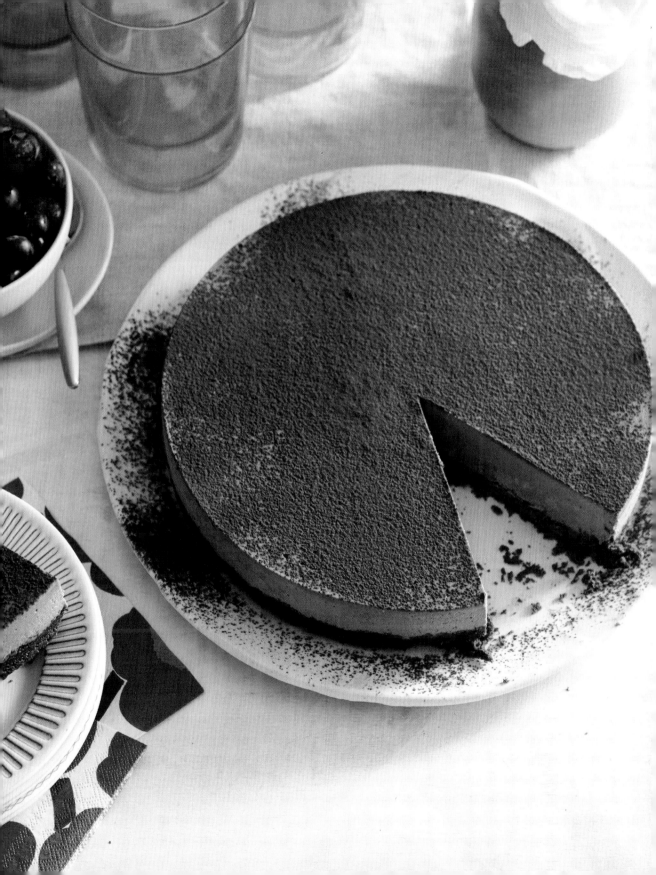

Chocolate-Coconut Popped Sorghum

In our house, we like to call this "baby popcorn," because when you pop sorghum, it looks like the tiniest kernels of popcorn you've ever seen. Just be aware that when popping sorghum, you'll get a large number of kernels that don't pop—more than with regular popcorn—so be sure to have extra on hand. If you're not a "sweet popcorn" person, consider drizzling your popped sorghum with a little olive oil, sea salt, and nutritional yeast for a "cheesy" popcorn-style snack.

SERVES 4

2 tablespoons extra-virgin olive oil

1¼ cups dried sorghum

½ cup bittersweet chocolate chips, melted

½ cup unsweetened shredded coconut

1 teaspoon flaky sea salt

1. Place a medium bowl next to your stove to remove kernels as they pop—sorghum burns quickly.

2. In a large, heavy-bottom saucepan with a lid, over medium-high heat, add a few (5 to 7) kernels of sorghum.

3. Cover, and wait until the kernels pop. (It's quieter than popcorn, so pay close attention.)

4. When the kernels have popped, remove from the heat, and add the oil along with the remaining sorghum.

5. Cover the pot, put on oven mitts, and shake to spread the grains. Let rest for about 30 seconds.

6. Return the pot to the heat.

7. Shake or stir frequently, until the popping slows down—you may notice some smoke, which is normal, but when the pot smokes, feel free to reduce the heat a bit.

8. As the kernels pop, strain them out with a slotted spoon (you don't have to get every single one) to prevent burning.

9. Once all the kernels are popped, drizzle with the melted chocolate, coconut, and salt. Toss to combine, then let cool (so the chocolate sets) before serving with plenty of napkins.

Crème Brûlèe

One of my favorite desserts—and I suspect yours, too—is much easier to prepare with an Instant Pot. Try serving your family this elegant créme brûlée after a weekend meal, and watch their eyes light up. Best of all, this sweet treat, rich in omega-3 egg yolks, is actually good for you!

SERVES 6

2 cups organic heavy whipping cream or coconut cream (save the thinner liquid from the can for something else)

6 large omega-3 egg yolks

⅓ cup monk fruit sweetener, divided

⅛ teaspoon sea salt

1 vanilla bean, scraped, or 1 tablespoon vanilla extract

1. In your Instant Pot, place the trivet on the bottom and add a cup of water to the pot.

2. In a large bowl, whisk together the cream, egg yolks, all the sweetener except 2 tablespoons, the salt, and the vanilla caviar scraped from the pod.

3. Pour the mixture into six 4-ounce oven-safe ramekins, and cover each with aluminum foil.

4. Carefully arrange three ramekins on the trivet, and place the remaining three ramekins on top of the first three—make sure the setup is sturdy.

5. Seal the pot, and cook on high pressure for 10 minutes. Let pressure release naturally for 15 minutes, then manually release.

6. Let cool to room temperature, then sprinkle with the 2 tablespoons sweetener.

7. With a blowtorch (or carefully, under a broiler), brown the brûlée topping until bubbly.

8. Serve, and enjoy.

Olive Oil Walnut Spice Cake

A sophisticated treat, this bread-like cake features warming spices and lovely herbal notes from olive oil. I like to pair a slice of this spice cake with a good strong cup of coffee. For an extra special treat, spread a little coconut whipped cream on your cake—it is positively decadent!

MAKES ONE 7-INCH CAKE

⅓ cup extra-virgin olive oil, plus more for greasing

2 cups almond flour

½ cup Swerve

2 teaspoons baking powder

½ teaspoon ground cinnamon

½ teaspoon ground nutmeg

½ teaspoon ground ginger

½ teaspoon ground allspice

¼ teaspoon ground cloves

⅛ teaspoon freshly ground black pepper

¼ teaspoon sea salt

2 large omega-3 eggs

⅓ cup coconut milk

½ teaspoon vanilla extract

½ teaspoon almond extract

1 cup chopped toasted walnuts

Coconut whipped cream, for serving

1. Grease a 7-inch oven-safe dish such as a cake tin or souffle pan with olive oil. Line the bottom with parchment, and set aside.

2. In the bottom of your Instant Pot, place the trivet and add 1 cup of water to the pot.

3. In a large bowl, whisk together the flour, Swerve, baking powder, cinnamon, nutmeg, ginger, allspice, cloves, pepper, and salt.

4. Add the eggs, oil, coconut milk, and the vanilla and almond extracts, and whisk until well combined. Fold in the walnuts.

5. Pour the batter into the prepared baking dish and cover tightly with aluminum foil. Set the baking dish in the Instant Pot on top of the trivet.

6. Cook on "cake" setting, then allow the pressure to release naturally for 15 to 20 minutes.

7. Carefully remove the pan from the pot, and let cool to room temperature.

8. Serve with the coconut whipped cream.

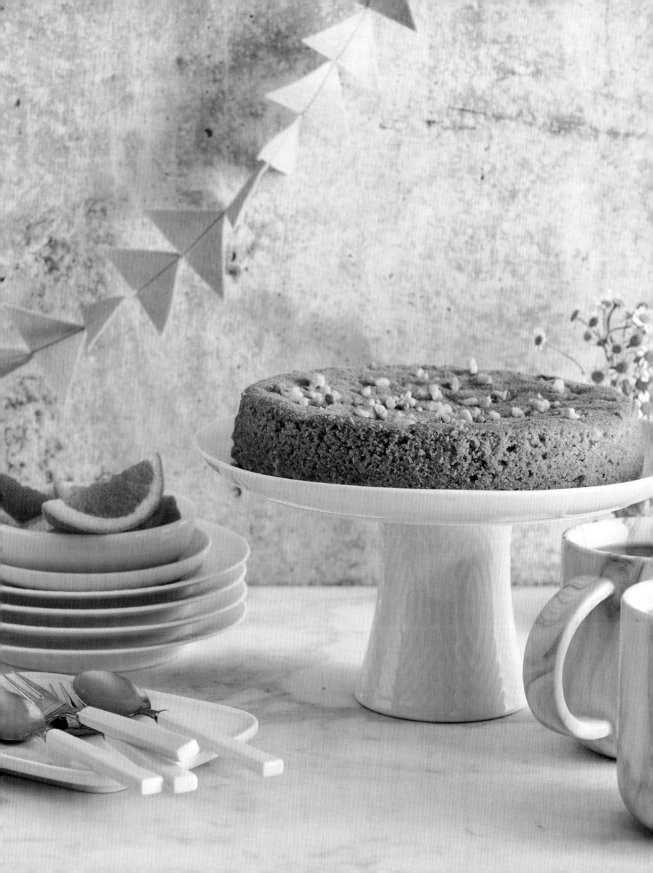

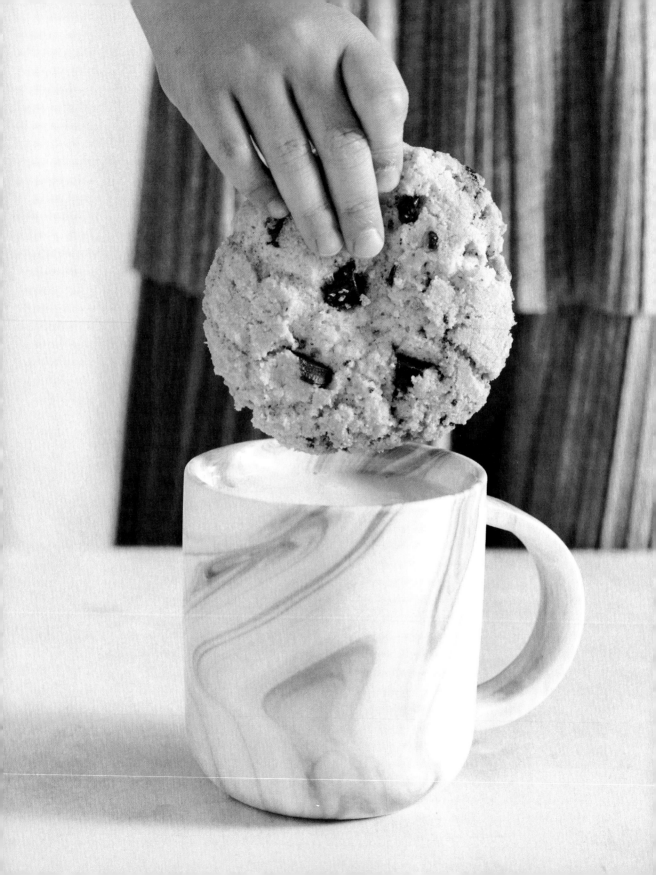

After School Classic Chocolate Chip Cookies

No one—not adults, not kids—wants to give up chocolate chip cookies for the rest of their lives! Luckily you can enjoy this classic treat on the Plan Paradox plan. Just a few easy ingredient swaps make these cookies as good for you as they are delicious. Pour yourself a glass of macadamia nut milk and drink away!

SERVES 12

1 ¼ cups blanched almond flour

½ cup coconut flour

½ tsp sea salt + more for sprinkling

½ tsp baking soda

½ tsp xanthan gum

¾ cup grass-fed butter or coconut oil

¾ cup Swerve

1 egg

1 ½ tsp vanilla extract

½ cup chopped bittersweet chocolate

½ cup shelled pistachios

1. Preheat the oven to 350°F. Line a sheet tray with parchment paper and set aside.

2. In a small bowl, whisk together the flours, salt, baking soda, and xanthan gum, and set aside.

3. In a mixer, or in a bowl with a hand mixer, whip together the butter or oil and Swerve until fluffy, about 2 minutes.

4. Add egg and vanilla continue to combine, for another minute.

5. Add chocolate and pistachios and fold to combine.

6. Roll the dough into twelve equally sized balls, and flatten slightly on the baking sheet. Sprinkle with salt and bake 12-18 minutes. Let cool before serving.

Keto Kids' Fudge Pops

I can't overstate how important it is to ensure your kids' eating revolves around vegetables, healthy fat, and some protein and not around carbs. With that in mind, we've developed this fudge pop recipe made with coconut cream and omega-3 eggs that's Keto-friendly and delicious. No kid can resist the clarion call of a fudge pop, and I am certain this healthy, homemade treat will soon become part of your regular rotation.

MAKES 6 FUDGE POPS

2¼ cups coconut cream, divided

¼ cup finely diced, extra-bitter dark chocolate (80% plus)

⅓ cup Swerve

2 large omega-3 eggs

1 teaspoon vanilla extract

1 tiny pinch of sea salt

1. In a small saucepan, whisk together half the coconut cream, the chocolate, Swerve, and eggs.

2. Cook, on very low heat, whisking constantly, until the mixture reaches a simmer.

3. Remove from the heat and whisk in the remaining coconut cream, the extract, and salt.

4. Pour the mixture into popsicle molds and freeze solid for 4 to 5 hours before serving.

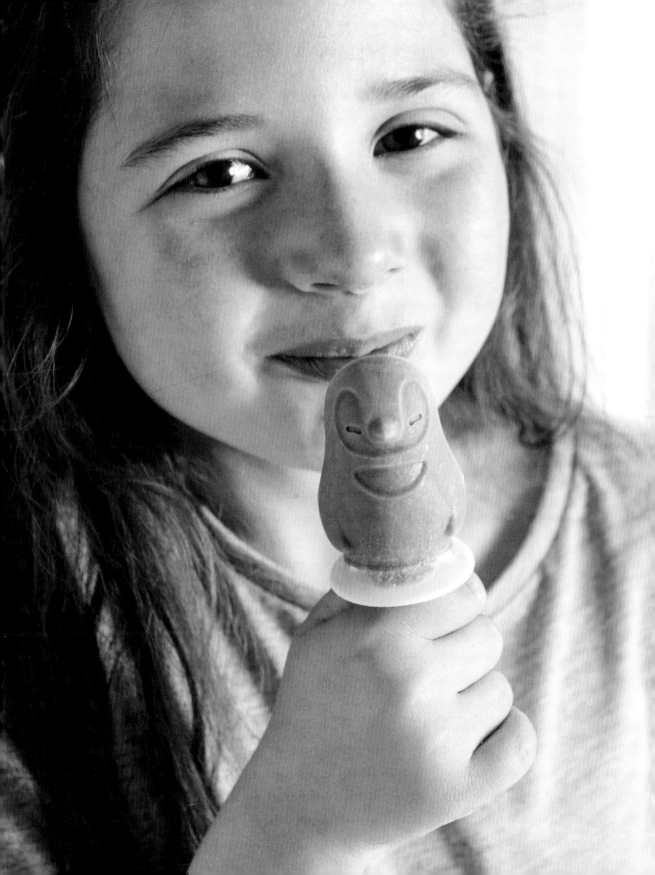

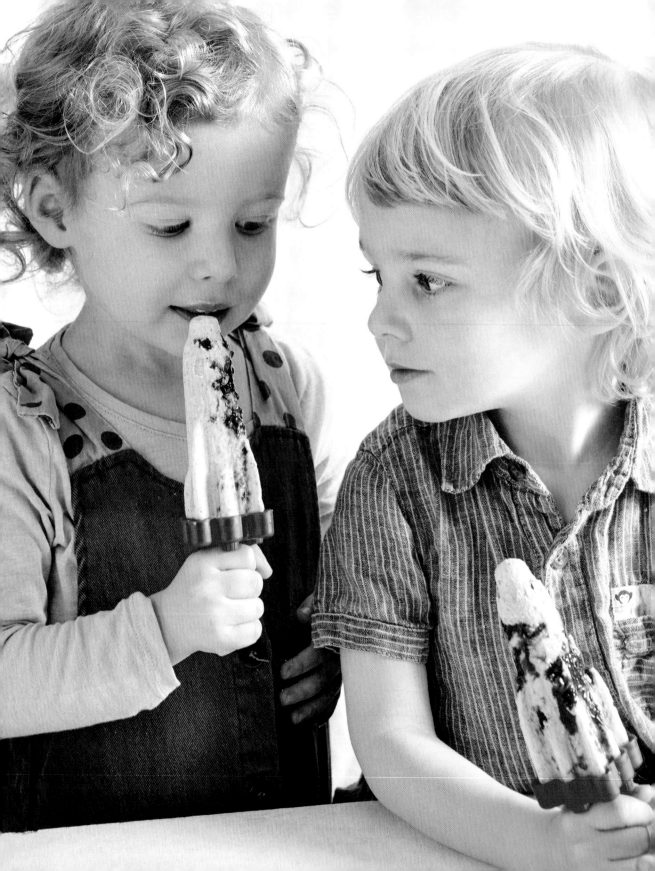

Almond Butter and Jelly Popsicles

These popsicles are my riff on the classic pb & j, minus the lectins! You can feel good about giving your little ones these icy treats made with almond butter, coconut cream, and homemade fruit jam. I recommend making a batch to keep on hand for snack attacks—they will keep well in the freezer for up to a month.

MAKES 6-8 POPSICLES

1 can coconut cream

½ cup almond butter

¼ cup monk fruit sweetener

⅛ teaspoon sea salt

½ cup Seasonal Fruit Jam (page 229)

1. In a high-speed blender, add the coconut cream, almond butter, sweetener, and salt, and blend until thoroughly incorporated.

2. Pour alternating stripes of the cream mixture and Seasonal Fruit Jam into the popsicle molds, and swirl with the popsicle stick or a skewer to create a "marbled" look.

3. Freeze at least overnight, before serving.

chapter twelve

Dips, Dressings & Condiments

Almost Classic BBQ Sauce

This tangy lectin-free barbecue sauce is a must-have when you're eating my BBQ Pulled Pork (page 145). Made with my Lectin-Light ketchup and a host of delicious (and antioxidant-rich) spices, this sauce is good enough to eat with a spoon!

MAKES ¾ CUP

1 tablespoon extra-virgin olive oil

1 sweet onion, finely diced

½ cup Dijon mustard

½ cup apple cider vinegar

3 tablespoons pomegranate molasses

¼ cup Lectin-Light Ketchup (page 220)

1 teaspoon turmeric

3 cloves garlic, crushed

1 tablespoon fresh, grated ginger

1 tablespoon coconut aminos, or fish sauce

1. Set your Instant Pot to sauté, and heat the oil.

2. Add the onion, and stir until the onion is caramelized.

3. Then add the mustard, vinegar, molasses, ketchup, turmeric, garlic, ginger, and coconut aminos, and switch to pressure cook. Cook for 10 minutes on high pressure, then manually release the pressure.

4. Switch the pot back to sauté, and simmer for 15 minutes.

5. If you're a fan of chunky barbecue sauce, use as is, otherwise, you can blend the sauce for 30 seconds until it's smooth. And that's it!

Lectin–Light Hummus

Homemade hummus is a heavenly thing, but most of the time it is also loaded with lectins. This pressure-cooked version is just what you've been waiting for—creamy, flavorful, and low in lectins, it's the perfect dip to pair with fresh veggies or spread on a sandwich or wrap.

1 cup dried chickpeas, soaked in 2 to 3 changes of water over 10 hours

4 cups water

1 teaspoon sea salt

⅓ cup tahini

Juice and zest of 1 lemon

2 cloves garlic

2 teaspoons smoked paprika

4 tablespoons extra-virgin olive oil

1. In your Instant Pot, add the strained chickpeas and water.

2. Cook on the bean setting (or at high pressure) for 20 minutes.

3. Let the pressure release naturally for 15 minutes. Manually release the pressure the rest of the way, then let the beans cool.

4. Drain the chickpeas, and transfer to the bowl of a food processor fitted with an S-blade.

5. Add the salt, tahini, lemon juice and zest, and garlic, and process until smooth. If too thick, thin with a little water.

6. Transfer to a serving bowl and fold in the paprika and 2 tablespoons oil.

7. Drizzle with remaining oil, and serve.

Serving suggestions: Serve topped with cubed avocado, drizzled with basil pesto, or topped with fresh herbs.

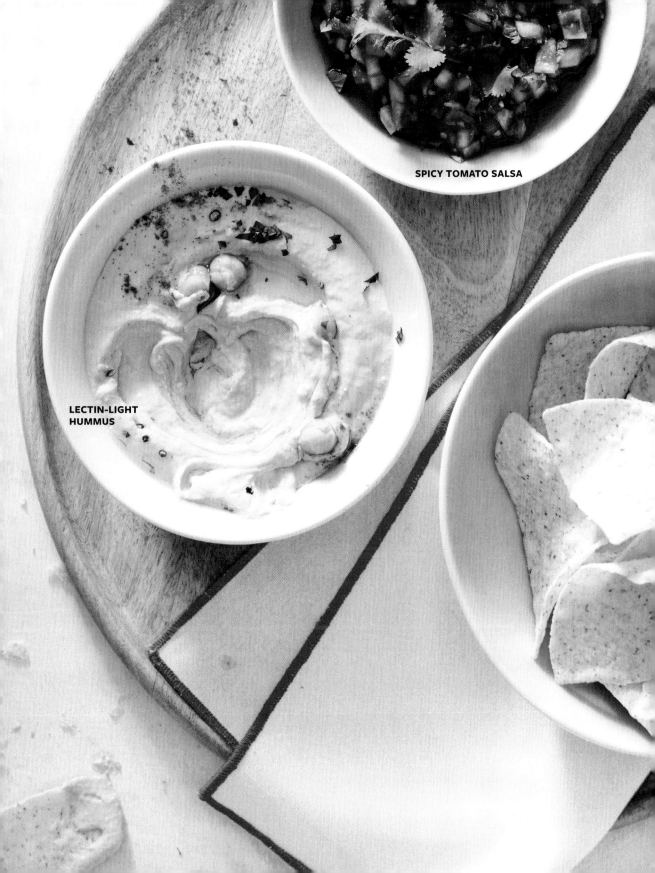

SPICY TOMATO SALSA

LECTIN-LIGHT
HUMMUS

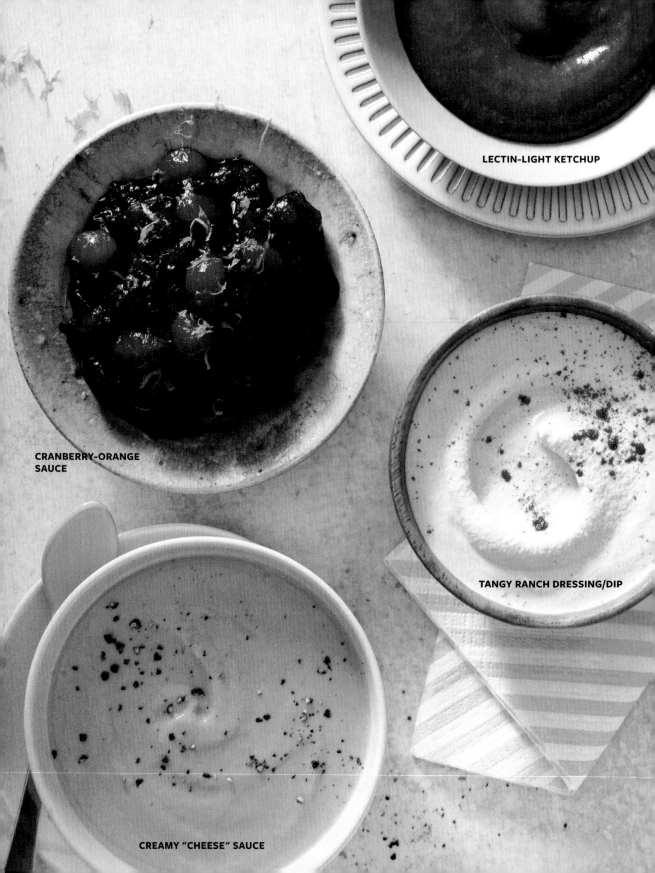

LECTIN-LIGHT KETCHUP

CRANBERRY-ORANGE
SAUCE

TANGY RANCH DRESSING/DIP

CREAMY "CHEESE" SAUCE

Tangy Ranch Dressing/Dip

This homemade ranch dressing is great drizzled on salads, as a dip for vegetables, or even spread on sandwiches. I recommend making a batch on Sunday and keeping a jar in the refrigerator so you have a quick way to add flavor to salads and bowls all week long.

MAKES 2 CUPS DRESSING

2 cloves garlic, minced

¼ cup flat leaf parsley, minced

2 tablespoons minced dill

2 tablespoons minced fresh chives

1 teaspoon freshly ground black pepper

½ teaspoon paprika

1 small shallot, minced

¼ teaspoon mustard powder

Zest and juice of ½ a lemon

½ teaspoon sea salt, plus more to taste

1½ cups plain coconut yogurt

Coconut milk, as needed

White wine vinegar, as needed

1. In a large bowl, stir together the garlic, parsley, dill, chives, black pepper, paprika, shallot, mustard powder, and lemon zest and juice.

2. Let the mixture mellow for 5 to 10 minutes, so the shallot looses its sharp taste.

3. Add the salt and coconut yogurt, and stir to combine.

4. Taste, and add more salt as needed.

5. Thin with the coconut milk and vinegar for a salad dressing, or serve as is for a dip.

* Keeps up to a week in the refrigerator.

Lectin-Light Ketchup

It's not a paradox! Tomatoes are full of lectins, but your kids don't need to give up ketchup, probably their favorite condiment, to thrive on the Plant Paradox. This pressure-cooked ketchup is even better then the jarred stuff at the store, and it's practically a requirement for my Pastured Chicken Nuggets (page 106). However, if you want to avoid even pressure-cooked nightshades, swap out tomatoes for sweet potato puree. You may need to add a little more vinegar to brighten the flavor, but the results will still be delicious.

MAKES ABOUT 2 CUPS

1 cup seedless, skinless tomato puree (from Italian tomatoes)*

⅔ cup water

2 tablespoons apple cider vinegar

1 tablespoon Swerve

1 tablespoon monk fruit sweetener

¾ teaspoon salt

1 teaspoon garlic powder

1 teaspoon onion powder

¼ teaspoon ground allspice

1 tablespoon tapioca starch

1 tablespoon water

Pinch of xanthan gum

1. To your Instant Pot, add the tomato purèe, water, vinegar, Swerve, sweetener, salt, garlic and onion powders, and the allspice.

2. Seal the lid and cook on high pressure for 5 to 7 minutes. Let the pressure release naturally.

3. Meanwhile, in a bowl, whisk together the tapioca starch and water.

4. When the pressure releases, turn the pot to sauté, and add the tapioca starch mixture and xanthan gum.

5. Let simmer and thicken, then cool. Store in an airtight container in the refrigerator for up to 3 weeks.

Dr. G's Tomato Sauce

This is my go-to recipe for all dishes—like pasta, meatballs, or pizza—that require tomato sauce. You can double the recipe to make a big batch and freeze half; it's great to have on hand when you need to pull together dinner in minutes.

MAKES 8 ½ CUP SERVINGS

4 tablespoons extra-virgin olive oil

1 small onion, minced

4 cloves garlic, minced

1 tablespoon minced fresh oregano

1 teaspoon sea salt

1 teaspoon freshly ground black pepper

2 28-ounce cans Italian tomatoes (peeled and de-seeded)

1 Parmigiano-Reggiano rind (optional)

1 tablespoon coconut aminos

1. Set your Instant Pot to sauté, and heat the oil.

2. Add the onion, garlic, oregano, salt, and pepper, and cook for 3 to 4 minutes, stirring occasionally, until the onion is tender and fragrant.

3. Then add the tomatoes and rind, seal the lid, and bring to high pressure. Cook for 45 minutes, then do a natural pressure release and open the lid.

4. Remove the rind, and add the coconut aminos.

5. Taste, and adjust the seasoning as needed.

6. Use immediately, or store in an airtight container and freeze for up to 6 months.

Caesar Salad Dressing/Dip

My spin on this popular dressing includes pine nuts and coconut yogurt, both of which make the dressing especially creamy. It does double-duty as a salad dressing or dip, great for lunch boxes with some cut-up vegetables, like asparagus spears, carrots, and celery.

MAKES 1 ½ CUPS

½ cup pine nuts, soaked in water overnight

Juice of ½ a lemon

1 clove garlic, crushed

1 teaspoon Worcestershire sauce or 2 teaspoons coconut aminos

1½ teaspoon anchovy paste (omit for vegan)

1½ teaspoons Dijon mustard

1 cup coconut yogurt

⅓ cup finely grated Parmigiano-Reggiano or nutritional yeast

1 teaspoon freshly ground black pepper

1. In the bowl of a food processor fitted with an S-blade (or a high-speed blender), add the strained pine nuts, lemon juice, garlic, Worcestershire sauce, anchovy paste, and mustard, and pulse until a smooth paste is formed.

2. Transfer to a bowl, and whisk in the yogurt, Parmigiano-Reggiano, and pepper.

3. Thin with water to make a dressing for salad, or serve as is for a dip.

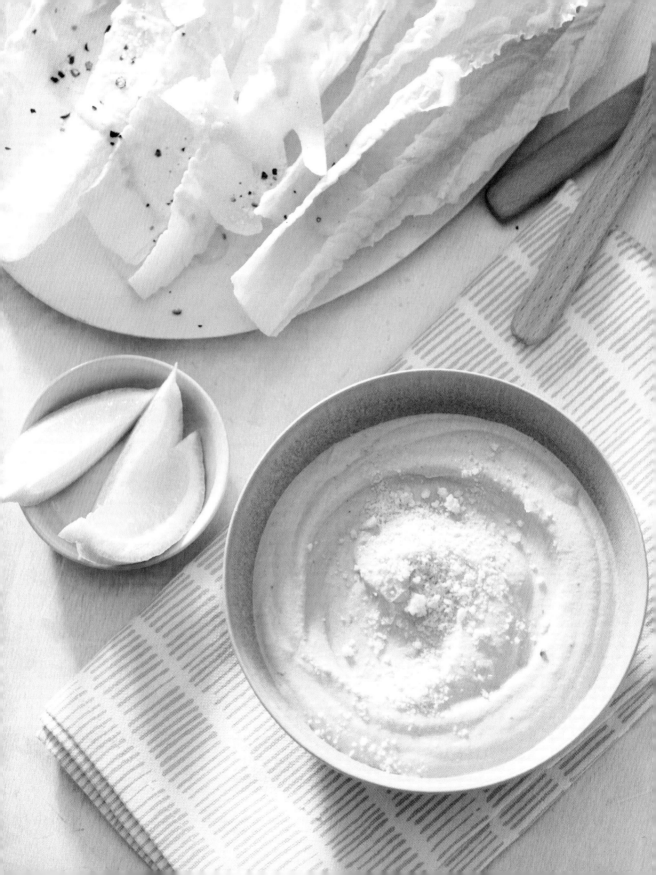

Sesame-Miso Dressing

I love the flavor of miso, which is a fermented soybean paste that's full of gut-friendly probiotics. Paired with the rich, buttery flavors of tahini (sesame paste) and sesame oil and brightened up with lemon juice, this is one of those recipes you will quickly memorize and find yourself making over and over again.

MAKES 1 CUP

⅓ cup miso paste

¼ cup tahini

Juice of 1 lemon

2 tablespoons sesame oil

1 tablespoon Dijon mustard

2 tablespoons rice wine vinegar

2 tablespoons yacon syrup or monk fruit sweetener

2 tablespoons coconut aminos

1. In a large bowl, whisk all of the ingredients together until well emulsified.

2. Taste, and add salt if needed.

3. Thin with water to dressing consistency, fold in coconut yogurt to make a dip, or use as a marinade for meat, seafood, or tempeh.

Spicy Tomato Salsa

I know, I know—salsa in a pressure cooker? It might seem crazy, but pressure cooking the tomatoes and jalapenos that are the stars of this salsa makes them safe to eat—and the flavor remains incredible! I like to use a good amount of garlic, onion, and jalapeno here, but feel free to customize to accommodate your family's taste buds.

MAKES 3 CUPS

1 28-ounce can crushed San Marzano tomatoes

1 large onion, finely minced

¼ cup peeled, seeded, and minced jalapeño peppers

2 tablespoons red wine vinegar

4 cloves garlic, minced

1 teaspoon sea salt

1 teaspoon cumin

¼ cup cilantro leaves, minced (optional)

1. In your Instant Pot, combine all of the ingredients except the cilantro leaves and cook for 20 minutes on high pressure.

2. Use a natural release to release the pressure, and allow to cool completely.

3. Taste, and adjust the seasoning as needed, then transfer to a serving dish.

4. Add cilantro if using, and serve, or transfer to an airtight container and freeze for up to 6 months.

Creamy "Cheese" Sauce

The "cheese" in this sauce is made from soaked macadamia or pine nuts; when blended, they provide a delicious, lush base with a texture that mimics melted cheese. As pine nuts can be pricey, try looking for them at Trader Joe's or Costco and buy in bulk for the best possible deal.

MAKES 2 CUPS (16 2 TBSP SERVINGS)

2 cups raw macadamia nuts or pine nuts soaked 4 to 10 hours in water

¼ cup tahini

½ cup nutritional yeast

Zest and juice of 1 lemon

1 teaspoon smoked paprika

1 teaspoon garlic powder

1 teaspoon onion powder

1 teaspoon freshly ground white pepper

1 teaspoon coconut aminos or sea salt

1. Thoroughly strain the soaked macadamia nuts, and discard the soaking water.

2. In the bowl of a food processor fitted with an S-blade, or a high-speed blender, add the nuts, tahini, yeast, zest and lemon juice, paprika, garlic and onion powders, white pepper, and coconut aminos, and pulse until gritty and well combined, then process until smooth—it takes longer than you think it will.

3. If needed, add water, a tablespoon at a time, until you reach a desired creamy consistency.

4. When the mixture is creamy and smooth, taste, and adjust the seasoning as needed.

5. Store in an airtight container in the refrigerator for up to 1 week.

Cranberry-Orange Sauce

This is the cranberry sauce that graces our family table at Thanksgiving, and we always try to make more than enough for one meal. Try spreading a generous portion on my Cranberry-Orange Breakfast Bread (page 98) as well as those delicious post-holiday Thanksgiving Sandwiches (page 163).

2 cups fresh cranberries

¼ cup water

¾ cup Swerve or monk fruit sweetener

Zest of 1 orange

1. In your Instant Pot, add the cranberries and water. Stir, and seal the pot.

2. Pressure cook on high for 1 minute, then let the pressure release naturally for 8 to10 minutes.

3. Vent manually the rest of the way, then open lid and switch to sauté.

4. Add the Swerve or sweetener and and orange zest, and cook, stirring, until the sauce is thickened.

5. Serve warm or cold.

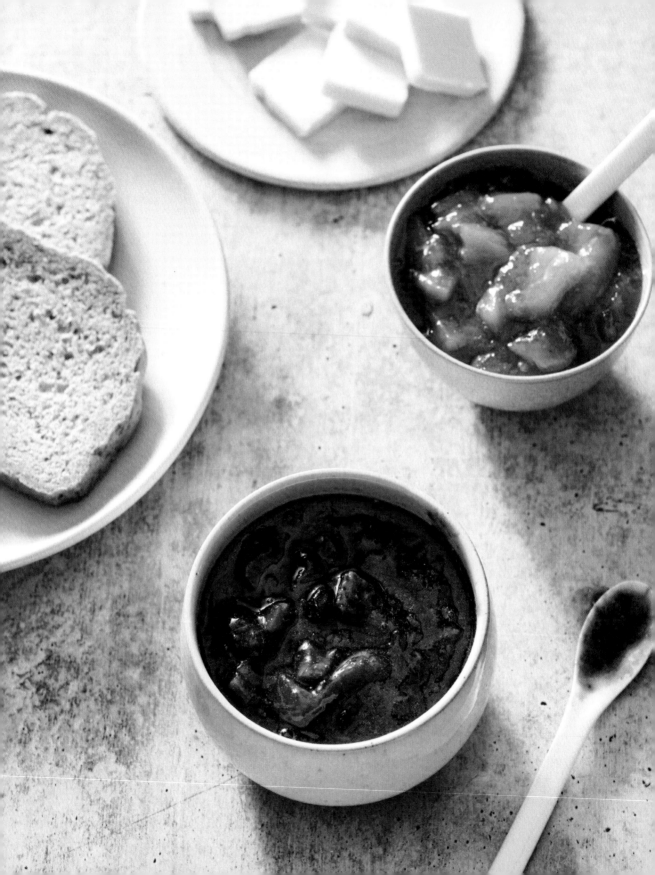

Seasonal Fruit Jam

Here is a simple and delicious fruit jam your kids will love, but unlike commercially prepared jams, it's free of sugar and light on lectins. Make sure to use fresh, in season fruit to keep the lectin content as minimal as possible.

MAKES ABOUT 3 CUPS, 15 TO 20 SERVINGS

2 cups peeled, seeded in-season fruit (cut into small chunks if large)*

1 cup Swerve

½ cup water

Juice of ½ a lemon

3 tablespoons tapioca starch

2 tablespoons water

Consider using strawberries, raspberries, peaches, blueberries, pears, apples, or figs, depending on season.

1. To your Instant Pot, add the fruit, Swerve, water, and lemon juice. Let the mixture rest for 10 minutes to draw liquid from the fruit.

2. Cook on high pressure for 1 minute, then let naturally release for 15 minutes. Switch to sauté.

3. In a separate bowl, combine the tapioca starch and water to form a slurry

4. Remove the lid (it *should* look soupy inside), and add the slurry.

5. Sauté, stirring and breaking up the fruit, until thickened.

6. Store in the refrigerator in an airtight container for up to 3 weeks.

chapter thirteen

Instant Pot Basics

Perfect Basmati Rice

If you must eat rice, I recommend choosing basmati, which is a grain that's been around for centuries. Just make sure to select *white* basmati rice, as the majority of lectins are in the hull (the brown part that's discarded). To make perfect fluffy basmati rice every time, all you need is 1 tablespoon extra-virgin olive oil, 1 cup basmati rice, 1¼ cups water, and a pinch of sea salt.

1. To make the rice, set your Instant Pot to sauté. Add the oil and rice, and sauté until the rice begins to look translucent at the edges.

2. Add the water and salt, seal the pot, and bring it to pressure.

3. Cook on high pressure for 6 minutes, then turn off the heat and release pressure naturally for 10 minutes. Manually release the rest of the way.

4. For bonus points, let the rice cool completely to allow more resistant starches to form, and reheat before cooking.

Pressure Cooker Beans

When cooking beans, I suggest soaking them in water for at least 6 to 8 hours (total) before cooking, and changing the water a few times during that period. It's not a necessary step for cooking tender beans, but it's 100 percent necessary for cutting down on lectins, so I wouldn't skip it, unless you're cooking lentils. Those, unfortunately, get mushy when they're soaked and then pressure cooked.

1. Once your beans are soaked, rinse them well, then place the them in your Instant Pot, along with any seasonings you plan on using. Add enough water to make sure the beans are completely submerged by at least 2 inches.*

2. Cook them on "Manual" or "Pressure Cook" mode at high pressure—I find this produces more consistent results than cooking on "Bean/Chili" mode. For cooking times, refer to the chart below.

3. When your beans have finished cooking, let the pressure on your Instant Pot release naturally for 10 minutes, before manually releasing the pressure the rest of the way. Then, drain any water, and serve, or use in the dish of your choice.

TYPE OF BEAN	COOK TIME
Black	25 minutes (35 unsoaked)
Pinto	20 minutes (30 unsoaked)
Lima	**15 minutes (25 unsoaked)**
Chickpeas (garbanzo beans)	**20 minutes (35 unsoaked)**
Lentils	**15 minutes unsoaked**
Navy	**30 minutes (40 unsoaked)**
Kidney	**30 minutes (40 unsoaked)**
Adzuki	**15 minutes (30 unsoaked)**

As a rule of thumb, use two cups of water for every one cup of lentils. If for some reason you are using unsoaked beans, use 8 cups of water for every 1 cup of unsoaked beans.

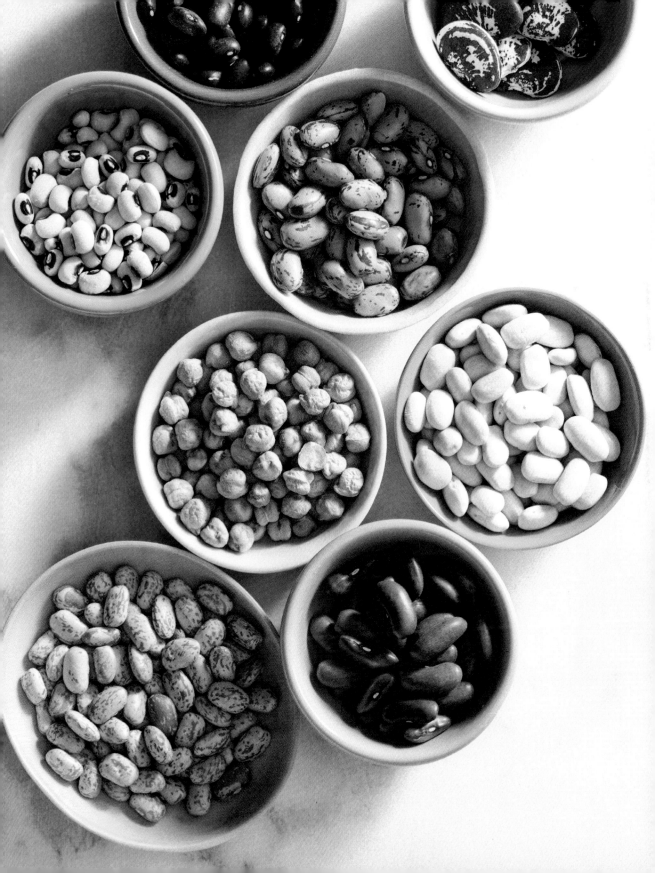

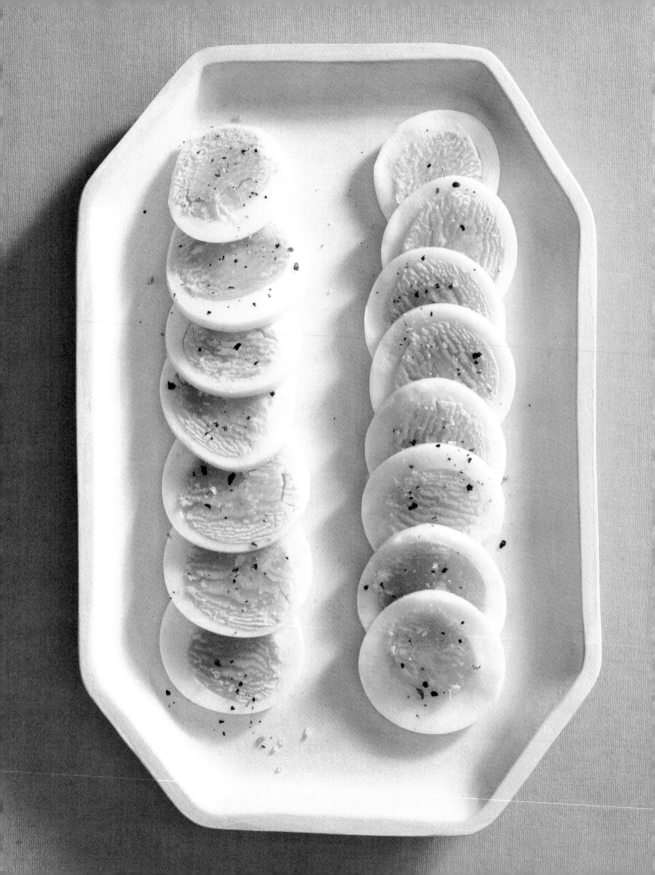

Pressure Cooker Hard-Boiled Eggs

Making hard boiled eggs in your Instant Pot is easy! I like to use a technique I call the 3 x 5 method, which involves cooking the eggs for five minutes, letting the pressure release for five minutes, and then cooling the eggs in an ice bath for five minutes. You will end up with perfect eggs every time.

1. To make eggs in the Instant Pot, place the rack in your pot, and add 1 cup of water. Carefully arrange the eggs on the rack, so they're not touching. Then, employ the 3 x 5 method.

2. Cook for 5 minutes at high pressure on manual mode.

3. Let the pressure naturally release for 5 minutes

4. Carefully transfer the eggs to the ice water bath, and let rest for 5 minutes.

5. Then, go ahead and peel the eggs—they should come out of their shells easily, leaving you with a quick, delicious, protein-rich snack you can enjoy any time.

"Baked" Potatoes

As you know, I'm not huge on white potatoes—they're part of the nightshade family. But if you must have white potatoes, I suggest cooking them in the pressure cooker to nix the lectins—and then taking it one step further, by cooling the potatoes completely and reheating them, which develops gut-nourishing resistant starch. To bake potatoes in your pressure cooker, all you need is a handful of potatoes (2 to 4 is good), 1 cup water, and a rack that fits into your appliance.

1. Scrub the potatoes until the skin is clean, then prick them a couple of times with a fork.

2. Pour the water into your pressure cooker, and arrange the potatoes on the rack.

3. Seal the pot, and cook at high pressure for 12 minutes (or up to 20 minutes for extra large potatoes).

4. After 12 minutes, let the pressure release naturally for 10 minutes. Then, release the pressure manually.

5. Let the potatoes cool to room temperature, then pop them into the refrigerator.

6. Let them cool all the way before heating them back up and using them.

"Baked" Sweet Potatoes

You can make perfectly tender "baked" sweet potatoes in a pressure cooker way faster than baking, which is great for a busy weeknight meal, or even a breakfast. And, of course, it will come in handy for the recipes in this book that include roasted sweet potatoes, which are a great binder. All you need is 2 to 4 sweet potatoes (small to mid-size ones are best), a pressure cooker fitted with a rack (it just makes life easier), and a cup of water.

1. Scrub the sweet potatoes until the skins are clean, then prick them a couple times with a fork and put them in the pressure cooker with 1 cup of water.

2. Bring the pot to pressure, and cook based on the times below. I find 15 to 20 minutes works for most sweet potatoes, but use the guide if you have a particularly large one.

3. Once cooked, allow the pressure to release naturally for 15 minutes, then manually release it the rest of the way before serving/using.

CIRCUMFERENCE AT WIDEST PART OF SWEET POTATO	COOK TIME
6 inches	15 to 20 minutes
8 inches	25 to 30 minutes
10 inches	**35 to 40 minutes**
12 inches	**45 to 50 minutes**

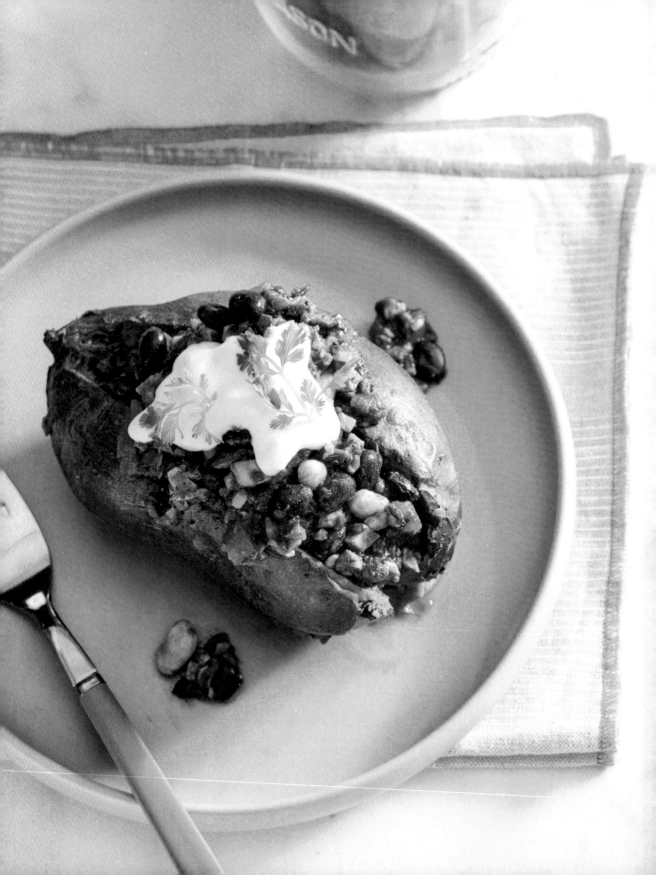

Pressure Cooker FAQs

There quite a few models of the Instant Pot, and this guide is not intended to serve as a replacement to the user's manual that comes with it—instead, it is designed to provide some tips, tricks, and hacks to make Instant Pot cooking simpler. Please read the user's manual that comes with your Instant Pot *before* you start cooking.

No matter which model of Instant Pot you have, your pot should come with the pressure cooker itself, the lid, the insert, or pot, and a wire rack that's handy for container-in-container cooking. If your model does not come with a wire rack, I suggest purchasing one from your local cookware store or Amazon—there are lots of Instant Pot-friendly options available.

Once you've read your user's manual, the best way to familiarize yourself with your new cooking gadget is to put it to use! I suggest starting with basic recipes like pressure-cooked beans or rice, as they'll give you a good sense of how your Instant Pot works. Along with the pressure-cooking settings (more on those below), make sure to try these other functions:

- **SAUTÉ:** The Instant Pot is great for browning food before pressure cooking—this really builds flavor for stews and other dishes. You can also sauté food before slow cooking, if using your Instant Pot as a slow cooker, or if you simply don't want to break out a pot or pan. In this book you'll also find some recipes that call for switching back to sauté after pressure cooking.

- **SLOW COOK/KEEP WARM:** Did you know you can actually use your Instant Pot like a slow cooker or crock pot? This setting comes in handy if you don't want another appliance crowding your kitchen. It's also great for keeping your pressure-cooked meals warm until your family is ready to eat.

- **YOGURT:** If you've ever been curious about making your own yogurt, this setting is for you. And great news—you can use it with coconut, goat, sheep, or A2 milk. All you need is the milk of your choice (I like to use coconut cream) and a high-quality probiotic supplement. Simply dissolve the probiotic supplement in the milk, switch to the yogurt setting, and let the Instant Pot do the rest! There are tons of guides on the Internet if you want to learn more about yogurt making in the Instant Pot.

- **CANCEL:** This button stops whatever you're doing and switches the pressure cooker to "off" mode. If you press it mid–pressure cooking cycle, you'll still need to wait for the pressure to release before opening the pot.

- **PRESSURE-COOKING SETTINGS:** Most of the recipes in this book use manual settings, as they are universal to all models of Instant Pots, but other settings include Meat/Stew, Bean/Chili, Poultry, Rice, Steam, Multigrain, and Porridge. Once you get the hang of the manual settings, you can try experimenting with these settings. (A word of caution: for some models of the Instant Pot, pushing the button for your desired setting more than once will change the temperature or the pressure of the setting, from low heat/pressure to high. Read your user's manual carefully.)

Pressure Cooking Basics

The basics of cooking in an Instant Pot are the same across the board. When you're ready to start the pressure-cooking process (after any seasoning or sautéing has been done), here's what you need to do:

1. Make sure there's AT LEAST a cup of liquid in your pot (or whatever amount is specified in your instruction manual).

2. Make sure your pot is not filled above the fill line marked on the inside of the cooking container (½ if you're cooking beans—especially unsoaked beans).

3. Double check that everything that belongs in the Instant Pot is *in* the pot (it's hard to stop cooking halfway through).

4. Put the lid on Instant Pot and twist to lock. Make sure the valve on top is switched to "sealing."

5. Hit the "manual" or "pressure cook" button and adjust the time up or down using the arrows.

6. Wait a few seconds, and the pot will start. It should beep and show "On" on the display screen. You'll notice the timer won't begin until the pot is pressurized, which can take 5 to 10 minutes.

7. When pot is pressurized, it will automatically start counting down the timer based on the cook time you've set. When cooking is done, it will switch to a natural pressure release (on some models, you'll notice and "L" in front of the timer at this point).

8. You can either leave the pot to automatically depressurize, or you can switch your pot to manual pressure release (see more about the pressure release settings below).

9. No matter which pressure release setting you select, wait until the float valve is completely dropped before attempting to open your pot, and beware of the steam that will be released as it is extremely hot and can easily burn you.

10. Once the pot is depressurized, open, remove food, or continue with your recipe.

Releasing Pressure

As mentioned, there are two ways to release the pressure on your Instant Pot: manua or natural (automatic).

- **NATURAL:** At the end of cooking, your pot will begin the automatic pressure release process, even if you don't vent the pot. If you notice an "L" next to your timer, and it is counting up rather than down, it is in automatic pressure release mode.

  If you want to naturally release pressure fully, you don't need to touch your Instant Pot at all after cooking—just leave it alone and the pressure will release. This can take up to 30 minutes depending on the recipe, so be patient. Your Instant Pot won't open otherwise.

  In this book, you'll notice that a lot of recipes call for a certain amount of time allowing for a natural pressure release followed by a manual release. This is to ensure the proper cook time for all ingredients in the pot while minimizing the minutes spent cooking.

- **MANUAL:** To manually release pressure (either right after cooking, or after a prescribed amount of time naturally releasing pressure), check that the vent of your Instant Pot is pointed away from anything sensitive to moisture or heat, and well out of the way of you or others.

Then, flip the valve on top of the lid from "Sealing" to "Venting"—you should notice steam releasing fairly quickly, letting out a loud hiss which may startle pets or children.

If you're manually releasing a recipe with a lot of liquid, you may also notice sputtering—this is normal, if a little messy.

No matter how you release pressure, once the float valve at the top of your Instant Pot has dropped, it is safe to open the pot. Always remember to open the pot away from your body.

Container-in-Container (or PIP) Cooking Made Simple

Many of the recipes in this book feature container-in-container (or Pot-in-pot, PIP) cooking. This is the term used for pressure-cooking a dish within a heatproof dish, rather than adding liquid directly to the dish and stewing. This method works well for foods like cakes and bread, egg dishes, and custards where you want to achieve a particular texture.

To use this method, look for heatproof containers that fit inside your Instant Pot, such as a 7-inch springform cake pan or 7-inch cake pan around 3 inches deep. You can also use silicone baking dishes, or even oven-safe stoneware or glass bakeware. Whatever dish you're using, make sure it is very well oiled with olive oil or avocado oil, for easy release after cooking. You can also line your dishes with parchment if you'd prefer.

When you're ready to cook, place the rack that comes with your Instant Pot inside the cooking pot, and add a cup and a half of water. Then, carefully lower your prepared container into the pot, so it's resting on top of the rack. One easy way to do this is to create a foil sling, and carefully lower it in. You can cook with the sling in the instant pot, and use it to lift the hot dish out when done. You can also use tongs, or specially designed gadgets available in cooking stores and online.

Instant Pot "hacks" to make your life easier

- **COOK MEAT FROM FROZEN.** I know that when I'm able to get a good price on wild-caught seafood or pastured chicken, I stock up and freeze some. And if you want, you can throw it right in the pressure cooker, frozen—just add 5 to 10 minutes of cooking time to whatever you're making to thaw food fully.

- **STACK YOUR FOOD.** If you're cooking food in ramekins, or even multiple container-in-container dishes with the same cooking time, go ahead and stack them, staggering them a bit. That way, you can make multiple dishes at once. A great way to do this is to use metal dim sum steamers or steamer baskets to create layers within your pot, or by buying multiple racks.

- **FREEZE MEALS IN ADVANCE.** Prepare and freeze uncooked meals in silicone molds that fit inside your instant pot. Then, when it's time to cook, just remove from the mold, dump in the pot, and cook. You can even cook right in the silicone mold, if it's oven safe.

- **USE YOUR DISHWASHER.** The rack and inner pot of your Instant Pot are dishwasher safe, and I find if you give them a good soak first, you can often drop them right in the dishwasher, no scrubbing needed.

- **FOR CRISP VEGETABLES, USE "0."** There's nothing worse than soggy vegetables, and sometimes the Instant Pot overcooks them. To make quick, perfectly steamed vegetables, put yours in a steamer basket, and cook for 0 minutes on high pressure—then release manually. The time it takes the pressure cooker to come to pressure is all you need to cook most vegetables.

- **BUY EXTRA SEALING RINGS.** The silicone rings are the first things to absorb smells, or to crack and break on Instant Pots, so it's worth keeping a few extra on hand. I've actually got one I use just for curries, since the smell works its way into the silicone almost immediately.

What Not to Do

- **DON'T BE AFRAID OF PRESSURE COOKING!** Instant Pots are not your grandmother's pressure cookers; if you follow the instructions that come with your Instant Pot, you don't need to worry about burns or explosions—electric pressure cookers are incredibly safe to use.

- **DON'T BE AFRAID TO USE MULTIPLE SETTINGS IN ONE MEAL.** You'll notice that many recipes start with sautéing and then transition to pressure cooking; this is a great way to build flavor.

- **DON'T FORGET TO PUT LIQUID IN THE POT.** Different sized Instant Pots require different amounts of liquid for cooking, but count on using at least 1.5 cups of liquid any time you cook with it—whether it's water, coconut milk, broth, or wine.

- **DON'T BRING YOUR INSTANT POT TO PRESSURE WITH THE VALVE ON "VENTING."** It should always be set for sealing when you're bringing food to pressure, or the pot simply won't pressurize.

- **DON'T UNDERESTIMATE TOTAL COOK TIME.** The cook time listed only reflects the time the food will cook in the Instant Pot—you need to account for any sautéing in the recipes, as well as the time it takes your pot to depressurize. That can be anywhere between 5 and 20 minutes, depending on the dish and the method.

- **DON'T BE TOO CONCERNED ABOUT THE "BURN" WARNING.** It's the most common error message you'll get, and it could happen for a few reasons:

  1. You could be using too little liquid. Try adding a bit more.

  2. You could have some sugars or burnt-on food caramelizing on the bottom of the pot. Add water to prevent this from happening.

  3. Your lid could be loose or your pot could be "Venting." Remove lid and reattach before using.

- **DON'T EXPECT THE SAME TEXTURE FROM BAKED GOODS.** Breads, cakes, and pancakes will come out a bit spongier than you might be used to, and more like steamed cakes, buns, or puddings. This is normal—and actually delicious.

Resources

For More Information Online

DRGUNDRY.COM

This is my personal website, where I post my thoughts, videos, and share breaking health news. It's also where you can tune into my weekly podcast, "The Dr Gundry Podcast." On the podcast, I give you the tools to live your best life, plus you'll get advice and insights from some of the greatest experts in the wellness industry.

DR. GUNDRY YOUTUBE PAGE
(https://www.youtube.com/drgundry)

Check out my Youtube channel for free cooking demonstrations and a whole library of recipes you won't find in any of my books!

Supplements

It's my firm belief that even if you have the most immaculate, health-promoting diet, you can still benefit from the right supplements. Why? Because modern farming practices, such as the use of pesticides, herbicides, and chemical fertilizers, have depleted our soil of nutrients and friendly bacterial populations. You simply can't get all the nutrients and micronutrients you need from food, because the food you eat isn't able to deliver those nutrients from the soil.

In my own life and in my practice with the thousands of patients I have seen, these are the supplements I recommend, because these vitamins and minerals are essential to our well-being, and the vast majority of us are deficient in them:

VITAMIN D

Even here in sunny Southern California, about 80 percent of my patients are vitamin D deficient when I first begin treating them, and that number is closer to 100 percent if those patients have an autoimmune disorder. This is a serious problem, because vitamin D plays an important role in helping your immune system to function, your bones to stay strong, and your beneficial intestinal flora and gut wall to be healthy. I recommend that everyone take at least 5,000 IUs of vitamin D3 daily, and if you have an autoimmune condition, make that 10,000.

B VITAMINS

B vitamins are key for protecting the inner lining of your blood vessels, and about half the population has a genetic mutation that prevents them from being able to convert folic acid and vitamin B12 into their active forms. To make sure you are getting enough B vitamins in a form that your body can use, I recommend taking methylfolate (the active form of folic acid), 1,000 mcg a day, and methyl B12 (the active form of vitamin B12), 1,000 to 5,000 mcg under your tongue each day.

GREEN PLANT PHYTOCHEMICALS

Your gut buddies love greens, but you have to take care not to take a greens supplement that contains lectin-rich grasses such as wheatgrass, barley grass, or oat grass. The supplements I recommend to lend you the vibrance of eating large amount of greens are:

- Spinach extract, 1,000 mg.
- DIM (diindolylmethane), an immune-boosting compound found in broccoli, 100 mg.

POLYPHENOLS

These phytochemicals protect plants from insects and sun damage, and they offer many benefits to you, including improved cardiovascular health and support of your gut bacteria. The polyphenol-containing supplements I recommend taking daily (you can choose one, or take a combination) are:

- Grape seed extract, 100 mg.
- Pine tree bark extract, 25 to 100 mg.
- Resveratrol (the polyphenol in red wine).

PREBIOTICS

Prebiotics are the substances that feed and nourish your gut buddies—they are the fertilizer that boosts the health of your internal garden. In addition to supporting your immunity, prebiotics will help to keep you regular. Good prebiotic supplements include:

- Psyllium husks, a teaspoon a day in water, working up to a tablespoon per day.

- Inulin powder, a teaspoon a day (the sweetener Just Like Sugar is primarily inulin).

LECTIN BLOCKERS

Remember, you can't avoid all lectins in your diet. For the lectins you do consume, it helps to have some lectin-fighting compounds in your system. These include:

- Glucosamine, which occurs naturally in the fluid that surrounds and protects your joints and serves a building block of cartilage, binds to inflammatory lectins and reduces pain. You can take one Osteo Bi-Flex or Move Free (both can be found at Costco) daily.

- D-mannose, the active ingredient in cranberries, is also an effective lectin blocker. Take 1,000 mg a day (divided into two doses of 500 mg each).

SUGAR BLOCKERS

To maintain healthy blood glucose levels, I recommend the following:

- CinSulin, a combination of chromium and cinnamon available at Costco, two capsules a day.

- Zinc, 30 mg.

- Selenium, 150 mcg.

- Berberine, 250 mg twice a day.

- Turmeric extract, 200 mg twice a day.

OMEGA-3S

Omega-3 fats are vital to the health of your gut and the health of your brain. In fact, half the fat in your brain—which is made up of 60 percent fat in total—is a long-chain omega-3 fat called DHA. Yet, in my ten years of seeing patients, nearly everyone is majorly deficient in these vital fats. Unless you're eating sardines or herring on a daily basis, you likely need to take an omega-3 supplement. I recommend:

- Fish oil, molecularly distilled and from small fish such as sardines and anchovies, enough to get 1,000 mg of DHA per day. Brands I like include Kirkland Signature Fish Oil (enteric coated, for no fish burps), OmegaVia DHA 600, and Carlson Elite Omega-3 Gems.

Acknowledgments

The Plant Paradox Family Cookbook could not have happened without the talents, and most importantly, the recipes developed at GundryMD by my collaborator and head chef extraordinaire, Kathryn "Kate" Holzhauer. Kate makes me and all my GundryMD YouTube segments look great and makes the food taste great, and now she's taken her talents to a new level! She not only designed and perfected so many of the dishes contained in this book, but also painstakingly tested them for ease of use. I think you will find out after just one recipe how easy it is to live a lectin-free lifestyle that promotes your and your children's health without giving up the tastes and textures you love. Thank you, Kate!

The team at HarperWave did it again. Thanks to my now longtime publisher Karen Rinaldi; Brian Perrin, director of marketing; and Yelena Nesbit, my new publicist. And of course, thanks to my dear editor extraordinaire, Julie Will, who lovingly beat me and *The Plant Paradox* into the major bestseller that has changed so many lives for the better, which, of course, fostered this book and all the rest. Thank you to Olga Massov for your collaboration, and thanks to the able team who helped create this beautiful package: Ellen Scordato and the team at Stonesong; photographer Evi Abeler, food stylist Julia Choi, and prop stylist Kristine Treviño.

And thanks to Omie Box, Appaman, and our little models, Logan, Bella, and Charlotte, for making the shoot fun.

All of my work is guided by my longtime agent and early believer, Shannon Marven, president of Dupree Miller; my attorney and longtime friend and supporter, Dave Baron; and my accountant Joseph Tames, who were able to corral all these disparate entities into a beautiful finished product.

As I said in *The Plant Paradox*, I cannot individually thank the entire 600-plus people at GundryMD who have made me and GundryMD.com the trusted source for health and supplement advice for millions of people daily, but I have to single out Lanee Lee Neil, who for the past year has daily, weekends as well, lorded over me and my brand. I couldn't have done it without you! And while away on maternity leave, Lanee was ably replaced by Christine Odonnell, who started the Dr. Gundry Podcast, providing even more helpful information from our great guests. Likewise, Amy Stanton and her team of publicists, including Rebecca Reinbold, Jessica Hofmann, Lauren Nelson, and the departing Lauren Newhouse at Stanton Company keep me and GundryMD in the spotlight daily. Thank you, all.

And speaking of "couldn't have done it without you," heartfelt thanks to my entire staff at The International Heart and Lung

Institute and The Centers for Restorative Medicine in Palm Springs and Santa Barbara, CA. As if things weren't busy enough before *The Plant Paradox*, wow, did you guys step up to the plate! Directed by Susan Lokken, my longtime physician's assistant, Mitzu Killion-Jacobo, my loyal team of Adda Harris, Tanya Marta, Cindy Crosby (who singlehandedly keeps the office afloat monetarily), Donna Fitzgerald, my daughter, Melissa Perko, Yessenia Parra, and of course the "Blood Suckers" led by Laurie Acuna and Lynn Visk.

Since this is a family cookbook, you will notice that my dedication goes out to our two daughters, Elizabeth and Melissa, their husbands Tim and Ray, and the grandkids, Sophie and Oliver. Elizabeth and Tim transformed their lives over the last two years with *The Plant Paradox*, and if they can raise their kids with it, so can you, dear readers!

Both this book and *The Longevity Paradox* were written while we were displaced from our home in Montecito, which was destroyed in the mudslides that killed 25 people, including our next-door neighbor. When they say home is where the heart is, nothing could be truer. Throughout it all, my wife Penny remained my "home" and continues to be so, even now that we have recently acquired a new place. Thanks Penny, again for being our family's anchor, and the home port I always long to return to from my travels.

Finally, like I said in *The Plant Paradox* and all my subsequent books, none of this would be possible without you, my patients and readers. Thank you for your trust in me and my team as we together try to maximize our collective knowledge, health, and longevity. And now, let's give our kids the best shot at great health for their long lifetime!

Endnotes

CHAPTER 1

1. Arizona State University. "Autism symptoms reduced nearly 50 percent two years after fecal transplant." ScienceDaily. www.sciencedaily.com/releases/2019/04/190409093725.htm (accessed July 17, 2019).

2. Chi, Liang; Bian, Xiaoming; Gao, Bei; Tu, Pengcheng; Lai, Yunjia; Ru, Hongyu; Lu, Kun. 2018. "Effects of the Artificial Sweetener Neotame on the Gut Microbiome and Fecal Metabolites in Mice." *Molecules* 23, no. 2: 367.

   Uebanso, Takashi; Ohnishi, Ai; Kitayama, Reiko; Yoshimoto, Ayumi; Nakahashi, Mutsumi; Shimohata, Takaaki; Mawatari, Kazuaki; Takahashi, Akira. 2017. "Effects of Low-Dose Non-Caloric Sweetener Consumption on Gut Microbiota in Mice." *Nutrients* 9, no. 6: 560.

3. Arizona State University. "Autism symptoms reduced nearly 50 percent two years after fecal transplant." ScienceDaily. www.sciencedaily.com/releases/2019/04/190409093725.htm (accessed July 17, 2019).

CHAPTER 2

4. Chia, Joanna S. J.; McRae, Jennifer L.; Enjapoori, Ashwantha Kumar; Lefevre, Christophe M.; Kukuljan, Sonja; Dwyer, Karen M. 2018 Sep 12. "Dietary Cows' Milk Protein A1 Beta-Casein Increases the Incidence of T1D in NOD Mice." *Nutrients* 10(9): 1291. doi: 10.3390/nu10091291

5. 6 University of Eastern Finland. "High vitamin D levels linked to lower cholesterol in children." ScienceDaily. www.sciencedaily.com/releases/2018/06/180607100942.htm (accessed July 17, 2019).

6. Agrawal, Rahul; Gomez-Pinilla, Fernando. 15 May 2012 "'Metabolic syndrome' in the brain: deficiency in omega-3 fatty acid exacerbates dysfunctions in insulin receptor signalling and cognition." *Journal of Physiology.* 590 (Pt 10): 2485–2499.

7. Mercola, Joseph. "Processed Foods Lead to Cancer and Early Death." Mercola. 27 February 2019. https://articles.mercola.com/sites/articles/archive/2019/02/27/health-effects-of-processed-foods.aspx

8. Ibid.

9. Ibid

10. Wang et al. 1998. "Identification of intact peanut lectin in peripheral venous blood." *Lancet* 352(9143): 1831-1832.

11. American Society for Microbiology. "Breast milk microbiome contains yeast and fungi: Do these benefit the infant?." ScienceDaily. www.sciencedaily.com/releases/2019/03/190301133843.htm (accessed July 17, 2019).

12. Mercola, Joseph. 27 February 2019. https://articles.mercola.com/sites/articles/archive/2019/02/27/health-effects-of-processed-foods.aspx (accessed July 17, 2019)

13. Smethers, Alissa D; Roe, Liane S; Sanchez, Christine E; Zuraikat, Faris M; Keller, Kathleen L; Kling, Samantha M R; Rolls, Barbara J. "Portion size has sustained effects over 5 days in preschool children: a randomized trial." *The American Journal of Clinical Nutrition*, Volume 109, Issue 5, May 2019, Pages 1361–1372, https://doi.org/10.1093/ajcn/nqy383

14. Simopoulos, Artemis P. 2 March 2016. "An Increase in the Omega-6/Omega-3 Fatty Acid Ratio Increases the Risk for Obesity." *Nutrients* 2016, 8(3), 128; https://doi.org/10.3390/nu8030128

15. Mercola, Joseph. 27 February 2019. https://articles.mercola.com/sites/articles/archive/2019/02/27/health-effects-of-processed-foods.aspx (accessed July 17, 2019)

16. The Endocrine Society. "Obesity speeds up the start of puberty in boys." ScienceDaily. www.sciencedaily.com/releases/2019/03/190325080418.htm (accessed July 17, 2019).

17. The Endocrine Society. "Chemicals in household dust may promote fat cell development." ScienceDaily. www.sciencedaily.com/releases/2019/03/190325080402.htm (accessed July 17, 2019).

18. Mercola, Joseph. 27 February 2019. https://articles.mercola.com/sites/articles/archive/2019/02/27/health-effects-of-processed-foods.aspx (accessed July 17, 2019)

19. Mellanby, May; Pattison, C. Lee. "Remarks on The Influence of a Cereal-Free Diet Rich in Vitamin D And Calcium on Dental Caries In Children." *British Medical Journal.* 1932 Mar 19; 1(3715): 507-510. doi: 10.1136/bmj.1.3715.507

20. Keeley, Jennifer. Michael Fields Agricultural Institute. 2004. "Case Study: Appleton Central Alternative Charter High School's Nutrition and Wellness Program." https://www.sustainlv.org/one/wp-content/uploads/Appleton-school-food-study.pdf (accessed July 17, 2019).

21. Simopoulos, Artemis P. 2 March 2016.

22. Simopoulos, ibid.

23. Sheppard, Kelly W.; Cheatham, Carol L. 2018. "Omega-6/omega-3 fatty acid intake of children and older adults in the U.S.: dietary intake in comparison to current dietary recommendations and the Healthy Eating Index." *Lipids in Health and Disease* 2016, 17 (43), https://doi.org/10.1186/s12944-018-0693-9

24. Keeley, Jennifer; Michael Fields Agricultural Institute. 2004.

25. Ozonoff, Sally; Young, Gregory S.; Carter, Alice; Messinger, Daniel; Yirmiya, Nurit; Zwaigenbaum, Lonnie; Bryson, Susan; Carver, Leslie J.; Constantino, John N.; Dobkins, Karen; Hutman, Ted; Iverson, Jana M.; Landa, Rebecca; Rogers, Sally J.; Sigman, Marian; Stone, Wendy L. "Recurrence Risk for Autism Spectrum Disorders: A Baby Siblings Research Consortium Study." *Pediatrics* 2011; 128(3)

26. Ibid.

27. West T, Atzeva M, Holtzman DM. "Pomegranate polyphenols and resveratrol protect the neonatal brain against hypoxic-ischemic injury." *Dev Neurosci*. 2007; 29(4-5): 363-72.

28. Barcelona Institute for Global Health (ISGlobal). "Maternal diet during pregnancy may modulate the risk of ADHD symptoms in children: Association found between omega-6:omega-3 ratio in the umbilical cord and the appearance of ADHD symptoms." ScienceDaily. www.sciencedaily.com/releases/2019/03/190328080410. htm (accessed July 17, 2019).

29. Ibid.

30. Cohen, Juliana F.W.; Rifas-Shiman, Sheryl L.; Young, Jessica; Oken, Emily. "Associations of Prenatal and Child Sugar Intake With Child Cognition." *American Journal of Preemptive Medicine* June 2018; 54(6); 727-735. DOI: https://doi. org/10.1016/j.amepre.2018.02.020

31. Cohen, Juliana F.W.; Rifas-Shiman, Sheryl L.; Young, Jessica; Oken, Emily. "Associations of Prenatal and Child Sugar Intake With Child Cognition." *American Journal of Preemptive Medicine* June 2018; 54(6); 727-735. DOI: https://doi. org/10.1016/j.amepre.2018.02.020

32. Chiu, Yu-Han; Williams, Paige L.; Gillman, Matthew W. "Association Between Pesticide Residue Intake From Consumption of Fruits and Vegetables and Pregnancy Outcomes Among Women Undergoing Infertility Treatment With Assisted Reproductive Technology" January 2018. *JAMA Intern Med*. 2018; 178(1): 17-26. Doi: 10.1001/jamainternmed.2017.5038

33. Roy, Priyanka; Phukan, Pranay Kumar; Changmai, Debojit; Boruah, Surajeet. "Pesticides, insecticides and male infertility" *Int J Reprod Contracept Obstet Gynecol* 2017; 6: 3387-91.

34. Ibid.

35. Sherry, C.L.; Oliver, J.S.; Marriage, B.J. "Docosahexaenoic acid supplementation in lactating women increases breast milk and plasma docosahexaenoic acid concentrations and alters infant omega 6:3 fatty acid ratio." *Prostaglandins, Leukotrienes and Essential Fatty Acids* 95 (2015) 63–69.

36. American Society for Microbiology. "Breast milk microbiome contains yeast and fungi: Do these benefit the infant?." ScienceDaily. www.sciencedaily.com/ releases/2019/03/190301133843.htm (accessed July 17, 2019).

CHAPTER 3

37. Nicklett, Emily J.; Kadell, Andria R. "Fruit and vegetable intake among older adults: a scoping review." *Maturitas* 75, 4 (2013): 305-12. doi:10.1016/j. maturitas.2013.05.005

38. Jiang, Y; Wu, SH; Shu, XO; Xiang, YB; Ji, BT; Milne, GL; Cai, Q; Zhang, X; Gao, YT; Zheng, W; Yang, G. "Cruciferous vegetable intake is inversely correlated with circulating levels of proinflammatory markers in women." *J Acad Nutr Diet* 2014 May; 114(5): 700-8.e2. doi: 10.1016/j.jand.2013.12.019.

39. Sheppard, Ibid.
40. Kwok, Chun Shing; Boekholdt, S Matthijs; Lentjes, Marleen A H; Loke, Yoon K; Luben, Robert N; Yeong, Jessica K; Wareham, Nicholas J; Myint, Phyo K; Khaw, Kay-Tee. "Habitual chocolate consumption and risk of cardiovascular disease among healthy men and women." *Cardiac risk factors and prevention* 2015; 101: 1279-1287.
41. Cuadrado *et al.* 2002. "Effect of natural fermentation on the lectin of lentils measured by immunological methods." *Food and Agriculture Immunology* 14(1) 41-44.
42. "Watch Your Garden Grow: Eggplant," University of Illinois Extension, http://extension.illinois.edu/veggies/eggplant.cfm, accessed on 10/12/17.

CHAPTER 4

43. Marshall University Joan C. Edwards School of Medicine. "Scientists tie walnuts to gene expressions related to breast cancer." ScienceDaily. www.sciencedaily.com/releases/2019/03/190328112514.htm (accessed July 18, 2019).
44. Fan, Xiajing; Liu, Hongru; Liu, Miao; Wang, Yuanyuan; Qiu, Li; Cui, Yanfen. "Increased utilization of fructose has a positive effect on the development of breast cancer." *PeerJ.* 2017; 5:e3804. 2017 Sep 27. doi:10.7717/peerj.3804

Index

Note: Page numbers in *italic* refer to photos.

About the Author

STEVEN R. GUNDRY, MD, is a cum laude graduate of Yale University, with special honors in human biological and social evolution. After grad- uating Alpha Omega Alpha from the Medical College of Georgia, Dr. Gundry completed residencies in general surgery and cardiothoracic sur- gery at the University of Michigan and served as a clinical associate at the National Institutes of Health. He invented devices that reverse the cell death seen in heart attacks; variations of these devices became the Medtronic Gundry Retrograde Cardioplegia Cannula, the most widely used device of its kind worldwide to protect the heart during open-heart surgery. After completing a fellowship in congenital heart surgery at the Hospital for Sick Children, Great Ormond Street, in London, and spending two years as a professor at the University of Maryland School of Medicine, Dr. Gundry was recruited as professor and chairman of cardiothoracic surgery at Loma Linda University School of Medicine.

During his tenure at Loma Linda, Dr. Gundry pioneered the field of xe- notransplantation, the study of how the immune system and blood vessel proteins of one species react to the trans- planted heart of a foreign species. He was one of the original twenty investigators of the first FDA-approved implantable left ventricular assist device. Dr. Gundry is the inventor of the Gundry Ministernotomy, the most widely used minimally invasive surgical technique to operate on the aortic valve; the Gundry Lateral Tun- nel, a living tissue that can rebuild parts of the heart in children with se- vere congenital heart malformations; and the Skoosh Venous Cannula, the most widely used cannula in minimally invasive heart operations.

As a consultant to Computer Motion (now Intuitive Surgical), Dr. Gundry was one of the fathers of robotic heart surgery. He received early FDA approval for robotic-assisted minimally invasive surgery for coronary artery bypass and mitral valve operations. He holds patents on connecting blood vessels and coronary artery bypasses without the need for sutures, as well as on repairing the mitral valve without the need for sutures and the heart-lung machine.

Dr. Gundry has served on the Board of Directors of the American So- ciety of Artificial Internal Organs and was a founding board member and treasurer of the International Society of Minimally Invasive Car- diothoracic Surgery. He also served two successive terms as president of the Board of Directors of the American Heart Association, Desert Division. Dr. Gundry has been elected a fellow of the American College of Surgeons, the American College of Cardiology, the American Surgi- cal Association, the American Academy of Pediatrics, and the College of Chest Physicians. He has served numerous times as an abstract re- viewer for the American Heart Association annual meetings. The author of more than three hundred articles, chapters, and abstracts in peer-reviewed journals on surgical, immunologic, genetic, nutritional, and lipid investigations, he has also operated in more than thirty countries, including on multiple charitable missions.

In 2000, inspired by the stunning reversal of coronary artery disease in an "inoperable" patient by using a combination of dietary changes and nutriceutical supplements, Dr. Gundry changed the arc of his ca- reer. An obese chronic diet failure himself, he adapted his Yale University thesis to design a diet based on evolutionary coding and the interaction of our ancestral microbiome, genes, and environment. Fol- lowing this program enabled him to reverse his own numerous medical problems. In the process, he effortlessly lost seventy pounds and has kept them off for seventeen years. These discoveries led him to estab- lish the International Heart and Lung Institute—and, as part of it, the Center for Restorative Medicine—in Palm Springs and Santa Barbara, California. There he has devoted his research and clinical practice to the dietary and nutriceutical reversal of most diseases, including heart disease, diabetes, autoimmune disease, cancer, arthritis, kidney fail- ure, and neurological conditions such as dementia and Alzheimer's dis- ease, using sophisticated blood tests and blood flow measurements to maximize his patients' health span and longevity.

This research resulted in the publication of his bestselling first book, *Dr. Gundry's Diet Evolution: Turn Off the Genes That Are Killing You and Your Waistline*, in 2008. Following up on the success of that book, he has be- come one of the world's authorities on the human microbiome and the interaction between the gut, the foods we ingest, the products we use, and our physical and mental health and well-being. In recent years, more than 50 percent of his practice has been devoted to the reversal of challenging autoimmune conditions in patients referred to him by health professionals around the world. These findings resulted in the publication of the *New York Times* bestseller *The Plant Paradox* and *The Plant Paradox Cookbook*, as well as *The Plant Paradox: Quick and Easy* and *The Longevity Paradox*. *The Plant Paradox* has been translated into over twenty- five languages and has prompted worldwide interest in a lectin-free diet. Dr. Gundry has been named to America's Top Doctors for twenty- one years in a row by Castle Connolly, the independent physician rating company; to *Palm Springs Life* Top Doctors for fifteen years in a row; and to *Los Angeles Magazine's* Top Doctors for the last six years.

Dr. Gundry is the creator of the nutritional guidelines for the Six Senses Resorts and Spas worldwide and a senior scientific advisor to Pegasus Capital Advisors. He has been invited to lecture at both the Stanford and MIT Brain Summit meetings on the impact of the gut on brain health and its deterioration. In 2016, he founded GundryMD, his own line of nutriceutical and skin-care supplements.

Dr. Gundry's wife, Penny, and their dogs, Pearl, Minnie, and George, live in Palm Springs and Montecito California. His grown daughters, Elizabeth and Melissa, their husbands, Tim and Ray, and their children, Sophie and Oliver, live nearby.